"I wish *Sidelined* had been published when I faced some of my own medical issues! Salenger's goal is to empower women to get the most out of their healthcare, including how to overcome the gender bias that exists in the medical community. I refer to it constantly and have found it incredibly helpful. All women should have this essential book in their health library!"
    —ELISSA GOODMAN, best-selling author, *Cancer Hacks*,
    Holistic Nutritionist

"*Sidelined: How Women Can Navigate a Broken Healthcare System* is a game changer of a book for all women. I live in London where our medical system is different, but this book is an incredibly valuable resource—to all women everywhere . . . a revolutionary and publishing milestone. *Sidelined* offers a wealth of suggestions on how to get the most out of your healthcare. An important and necessary book that just might save your life!"
    —BRIX SMITH START, musician and author of
    The Rise, The Fall, and The Rise

"Enjoyable to read and meticulously researched, *Sidelined* offers profound insights into the unique challenges women face as they handle their healthcare. Salenger weaves together psychology, sociology, anthropology, medical history, current research, and personal narratives to help women better care for and advocate for themselves. This is definitely a book every woman (and every doctor) should read!"
    —JILL WARBURTON, PSYD., Berkeley California

"*Sidelined* is both a subtle eye-opener and a wake-up call. Subtle because intelligent and responsible women rarely see themselves as neglecting their own health. And yet, *Sidelined* describes how we often neglect ourselves and quietly put off medical and health care appointments so that we can tend to other people and other commitments before we take care of ourselves. A wake-up call because even in this new age of "enlightenment," women still face gender bias from the medical profession. Women continue to be patronized, our issues still sometimes considered emotional and hysterical rather than physical and substantial. *Sidelined* is a wake-up call to advocate courageously and confidently on our own behalf."
—JANET CONSTANTINO, M.A., MFT, Licensed Marriage and Family Counselor

"Even though *Sidelined* is a book for women, it's imperative that husbands, lovers, partners and the entire family take note of the issues Salenger describes. You'll find life-saving ideas, tips, skills and techniques that will impact someone you know and, of course, YOU! Salenger has done her homework for us – this is a book that should not be dismissed but should be devoured."
—NANCY FRIEDMAN, Founder, Chairman—Telephone Doctor Customer Service Training

SIDELINED

SIDELINED

How Women Can Navigate a Broken Healthcare System

SUSAN SALENGER

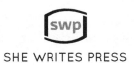

SHE WRITES PRESS

Published 2022
Printed in the United States of America
Print ISBN: 978-1-64742-401-5
E-ISBN: 978-1-64742-402-2
Library of Congress Control Number: 2021916462

For information, address:
She Writes Press
1569 Solano Ave #546
Berkeley, CA 94707

Interior design by Tabitha Lahr

She Writes Press is a division of SparkPoint Studio, LLC.

"I'm interested in women's health because I'm a woman. I'd be a darn fool not to be on my own side."

—Maya Angelou

CONTENTS

WHY DID I AGREE TO THAT?

Why This Book Matters

Scared, hungry, and half tranquilized, I watched while hospital staff wheeled me into the OR. I was furious at myself for consenting to have surgery I was confident I didn't need. Yet here I was, lying on a gurney, hooked up to IV tubes, surrounded by hospital personnel, and feeling vulnerable and foolish. I'll tell you about my operation in a bit—it went fine. This is not a story about tragedy.

But it *is* a story about how we, as women, manage—and sometimes mismanage—our healthcare. As a group, we're very conscientious about taking care of ourselves. We choose our doctors carefully, visit them more frequently than men do, try to keep up with all our tests, and stay on top of the latest health information.[1] At the same time, we sometimes inadvertently make decisions that can undermine our own health.

For example, sometimes there's simply no time for a routine checkup. It may be too hard to take time off from work, or there's no one to watch our kids. We may blame ourselves for getting sick and feel too ashamed and embarrassed to call the doctor, which can only make us feel even worse and more vulnerable. Or we may hesitate to get a second opinion because we don't want to hurt our primary doctor's feelings. After all, we don't want to be thought of as difficult, or worse, rude. We can get so caught up in our fears and our everyday lives that, by failing to seek timely medical care, we do ourselves a disservice. Then, should unanticipated consequences develop, we say to ourselves (as I did), "What in the world was I thinking?"

So why did I agree so quickly to have a surgery I felt pretty sure I didn't need? Why was I lying on that gurney? Thinking about it today, I realize I behaved just as passively as my grandmother did when she thought she was sick. She would phone my mother and, in a faint, weak voice, tell her she wasn't feeling well but didn't want to "bother the doctor." She wanted my mom to call for her. Why my mom's call wouldn't bother the doctor, I could never figure out. Later she would call back to find out what the doctor said. Even as a child, I understood she was lonely and needed contact with my mom. But, still, I wondered why that kept her from acting on her own behalf.

Looking back, I see how my behavior wasn't all that different from my grandmother's. She was too anxious, deferential, and insecure about calling her doctor; I was too anxious, deferential, and insecure to question my doctor and trust my gut instincts. Just like her, I became passive, and I acquiesced. After all, he was the professional.

My operation was exploratory. I called the doctor because I was experiencing unusual vaginal bleeding. At his suggestion, I had switched from one postmenopausal hormone to another that he believed would be more effective at protecting against osteoporosis. I had been taking the new hormones for just a few weeks when the bleeding began. Because I'm especially sensitive to medication and don't believe in medical coincidences, I was sure the new hormones were to blame. When I returned to the doctor, I insisted we switch back to my old regimen to see if the bleeding would subside. He vehemently disagreed, saying that none of his other patients had experienced bleeding from this medication and that vaginal bleeding can be a symptom of something much more serious. After doing some preliminary testing, he found nothing wrong and urged me to have exploratory surgery.

Despite my initial reservations that the surgery was totally unnecessary, I was so anxious that I might have a serious disease that I not only agreed to follow the doctor's advice, but I insisted the surgery be sooner rather than later. I could tell he was worried, and, because I'm a worst-case-scenario type, I was sure he was thinking of cancer. But I didn't even think to *ask* what he was thinking and, instead, rushed ahead to schedule it. At the time, I was a young woman with young children and, had he been right, he would have saved my life.

But he wasn't. The operation showed nothing wrong, and he agreed that I could return to my original hormones. As soon as I did—no surprise—the bleeding stopped.

And while I felt vindicated that my original conviction was accurate, I still felt bad for agreeing to the surgery, particularly given all the things that *could* have gone wrong. General anesthesia has inherent risks, and hospitals are rife with infections, some resistant to all antibiotics. In the United States, some reports say that there are at least two hundred fifty thousand iatrogenic deaths annually—deaths caused by the medical treatment itself. Since my surgery was elective, I could have waited at least a week or two, gotten a second opinion, and given myself more time to put things in perspective.

The surgery happened over thirty years ago. I was busy living my life, raising two young children, and running a business, so although I thought about it from time to time and wondered why I had agreed to it so quickly, I didn't really dwell on it. But then, after the kids grew up and I had some time for myself, I decided to take some anthropology classes at UCLA. For one of them, my final project was a study of women who had undergone hysterectomies. Since my surgery was also gynecological, it reminded me of my own surgery, and I became curious to see if any of the women in my study felt similar regrets. I learned that while some were very happy with their hysterectomies and said they felt much better afterward, like me, a few regretted their surgery: they, too, had agreed to surgery despite being unconvinced they truly needed it. And although my surgery was just exploratory, theirs were irrevocable, with permanent repercussions.

I was surprised at the degree of regret I heard because it seemed at odds with other things we know about how women manage their health. Besides being extremely diligent about our own health to-do list, we're also the medical gate-keepers for our families. We're the ones who traditionally encourage our husbands, partners, and children to seek medical treatment and follow through with their care.[2] In fact, we make approximately 80 percent of all healthcare-purchasing decisions in the United States. (A statistic, by the way, about which pharmaceutical companies are well aware. That's why so much of their advertising is directed toward women.[3])

But I was confused by the conflict I saw between the energy and thoughtfulness women put into their own health-care and the amount of regret they expressed to me about at least one major healthcare decision they had made. That's when I finally decided to sit down and write about it.

To help myself understand what I was observing, I needed to do some research. I reviewed academic studies about women, illness, and healthcare. I studied cultural commentators like Barbara Ehrenreich and women's health researchers like Laurie Edwards to see what they had to say. And I talked with more than forty women about their health. Everyone's experiences varied, of course, but a general pattern emerged: I found six common decisions women inadvertently make that undermine their health and their healthcare. In each of the chapters that follow, I discuss these decisions in detail, but here is a brief overview:

1. We put others first.

There's always so much else to do in a day! We have breakfast to make, children's lunch boxes to fill, sick parents and other relatives to care for, and perhaps a major presentation to deliver at work. There's just no time left to care for ourselves.[4]

2. We're too quick to defer.

One woman I met said, "Who am I to question my doctors? They're the professionals." I remember thinking that exact same thing when I agreed to my surgery. Some of us are afraid that we'll seem pushy. And when we're frightened, we certainly don't want to offend the people caring for us.

3. We blame ourselves for getting sick.

Another woman told me her illness was punishment for past behavior: "I'm sure my illnesses are total payback for all the people I've hurt during my life." Stress is another common scapegoat, and many blamed their illnesses on their inability to handle it. Dr. Donna Stewart found that 42 percent of the women in her research blamed their breast cancer on stress.[5]

4. We speak a different language than our doctors do.

Women and men speak differently to doctors. We tend to describe our symptoms more completely than men, and we explain how they affect us emotionally as well as physically.[6] This "female" conversation style can do more harm than good, since it can lead doctors to assume our problems are psychological rather than organic. Laurie Edwards describes a survey conducted by the American Autoimmune Related Diseases Association that found that of the thirty-seven million women who suffer from autoimmune diseases, 45 percent were labeled chronic complainers when they attempted to get an accurate diagnosis. It took some of them so long to find out what was going on that they suffered organ damage in the process![7]

5. We overlook the role of emotions in our recovery.

Although we focus on the emotional aspects of our illnesses when describing our symptoms, when it comes to recovery, we tend to take the opposite approach: we focus on the physical relief we're hoping for and neglect to think about the potential emotional ramifications that could affect our recovery. In other words, when we make our decisions, we look at only half the story and risk missing out on the bigger picture.

6. We're too quick to reach for a pill.

In 2017, *Consumer Reports* revealed that more than half of all Americans take an average of four prescription drugs daily, and that women are prescribed more drugs than men are.[8] We go to the doctor more often than men do, suffer disproportionately from chronic diseases and pain, and purchase most of our families' medications. That's why drug company ads target us.[9] And these ads are *very* successful![10]

This book explores in depth the serious repercussions of each of these behaviors for our physical and emotional health. As in my case, we may move too quickly and agree to treatment we don't need—or, by failing to speak up for ourselves, we may move too slowly and fail to get treatment we do need.

And here's a sad truth for you: every ninety seconds, a woman in this country will suffer a heart attack; annually, three hundred thousand women will die from them. But in a 2012 AARP survey, *only half* of all women who participated said they would call 911 after experiencing heart attack symptoms. Why? The main reasons were that they wouldn't want to bother anyone or have the paramedics see their messy house.[11]

In fact, so many women hesitate to call for help that the U.S. Department of Health and Human Services' Office on Women's Health developed a national public education campaign, "Make the Call, Don't Miss a Beat," to educate women to call 911 immediately if they think they are having a heart attack.[12]

Imagine *this* on your tombstone: "If only she had kept a neater house, she'd be alive today."

Why do so many of us take such good care of ourselves and our families while, at the same time, doing such a serious disservice, however unwittingly, to our own health?

Before I answer, I want to be clear: this not a blame-the-victim diatribe. I know that women are perfectly capable of handling their own and their family's healthcare. But I also know that we approach our medical care with preconceived attitudes, some of which are more productive than others. And I know that some doctors (male and female) approach us with their own preconceptions. *In The Kingdom of the Sick* (2013), Laurie Edwards explains that "deeply ingrained ideas about women . . . as weaker than men, as histrionic or otherwise 'emotional,' have had a profound impact on their ability to receive accurate diagnoses and appropriate care."[13]

My belief is that women have internalized some of these "deeply ingrained ideas" and that we've been conditioned by various historical and cultural factors to see ourselves as physically and emotionally vulnerable. It's important to understand where these "deeply ingrained ideas" come from, and that's why the last chapter lays some of them out in a brief historical tour. We begin with the attitudes toward women as far back as ancient Greece and go all the way up to today. From the belief of Hippocrates (the father of medicine) that gynecological disorders made women's bodies inherently pathological to the Victorian focus on "hysteria" to today's war on reproductive rights, women and their bodies have continued to be devalued and misunderstood.[14] And despite the fact that we make up over 50 percent of the workforce, we're still often told to stay in our place as mothers and caregivers. It's no wonder we might be reluctant to take time for ourselves or question our doctors' opinions.

My point is that women's attitudes toward themselves and their health don't exist in a vacuum, and part of my goal in this book is to help women become more self-aware about why we do what we do and how we make our healthcare decisions: ignoring our gut instincts, deferring to our doctors, blaming ourselves for our inability to handle stress, putting our own health behind the needs of our families and friends — these are the negative and potentially vicious cycles I want to help women recognize and break.

I know this is no easy task. In fact, what surprised me the most in doing this research was how many women said they had *never* previously discussed their health with anyone other than their doctors. I could hear how alone some of them felt. "After a while, people don't care," one woman explained. "They just think you're whining." For interview purposes, I put together some focus groups, and I could see how relieved the women were to discover other women — regardless of their particular illness — who were coping with similar issues of vulnerability, self-blame, and shame about being ill.

And that's another reason I wrote this book, to encourage conversation among women about their healthcare and the issues they face because of it. Illness can be a long and difficult journey to take alone.

Certainly not *all* women experience *all* of the issues listed here. Maybe you'll see yourself in only one or two of them. But whichever resonates, hopefully you'll find that understanding some of what underlies your decisions will make it easier to assess if you're on the right track as you think about your health.

But that's only the first step. Just as important is developing some strategies to avoid making decisions that go against your best interests. That's why each chapter includes tools to help deal with whatever is standing in your way.

Clearly women are a diverse group, and, for myriad reasons, the medical profession treats some women differently from others. For practical purposes, I have referred to women as a whole, without trying to divide us into subgroups. While I recognize this approach has limitations, it is beyond the scope of the material covered here to address the specific issues of each subgroup.

To protect their privacy, I have changed the names and locations of most of the women whose stories I recount. A few of the women specifically wanted me to use their real names.

I hope that if you recognize yourself in these pages and find the suggestions useful, your healthcare experiences will become more satisfying and productive. I want to ensure that when you think about your medical decisions, you'll never have to ask yourself, like I did, "What *was* I thinking?"

CHAPTER 1

"AFTER YOU"

Putting Others' Needs
Before Our Own

Desireé Daruma is a forty-year-old Filipina who moved to Boston with her two dogs after her eleven-year marriage ended in divorce. She suffers from lupus erythematosus, a chronic autoimmune disease that occurs when the body's immune system attacks its own healthy tissues and organs. Desireé has a very common way of thinking about the importance of her own health:

> It turned out the man I was living with was a habitual liar and a con artist who scammed people for money. Even though I was so stressed—I lost weight and my hair began to fall out—I stuck it out for six months because he needed my help to qualify for Medi-Cal and food stamps. He was making me worse, but I ignored my lupus flares and just did what I needed to do so I could get him what he needed.

Women can be so busy taking care of others that we often put off taking care of ourselves. "Doing our duty" and caring for other people is so ingrained, so much a part of us, that it seems as if it's in our DNA. Our responsibilities lead us to make excuses about why now is not a good time to call or go to the doctor. For example, we may say to ourselves, "There are only twenty-four hours in a day, after all, and how am I supposed to get my children off to school or finish that project at work?" "I don't have time to make a phone call, let alone fill the prescriptions the doctor might say I need. Plus, if my family sees I'm not feeling well, they'll be upset and want to help take care of me. Then I've become a bother." "Even worse, what if the reason for my visit turns out to be a false alarm? How embarrassing! My doctors might blame me for wasting their time."[1]

So we tell ourselves and others, "It's nothing. No worries." After all, we don't feel *that* bad, and we don't want to take doctors away from someone who *really* needs them.[2]

A recent survey conducted by *Healthy Women* and *Working Mother* magazines showed where women put themselves in a hierarchy of who they should care for first:[3]

❖ Children
❖ Pets
❖ Elder relatives
❖ Spouses or significant others
❖ Themselves

In all, 78 percent of the women surveyed said they put off taking care of themselves because they're so busy taking care of others.

Eighty-two percent of women in the United States do most of the health-related research for their kids.

Eighty-six percent schedule the majority of the health care appointments for their kids.

Seventy-two percent arrange for the payment of the majority of the bills for their kids' health care.[4]

Delaying or ignoring our heath care comes with serious risks: For example, women do not recover from cardiovascular disease as well as men do. We experience greater disability and have a higher rate of complications and early death after an acute coronary event. Regardless, fewer of us attend cardiac rehabilitation programs despite their proven benefits.

Why Women Put Themselves Second

As women, we think of many reasons to put our health last. And they all make perfect sense to us at the time we think them. But they may do us a serious disservice.

We're Busy

Dr. Michelle DiGiacomo, from the University of Technology Sydney in Australia, and her colleagues wondered if caregiving responsibilities caused women to let their own health slide. They gave questionnaires to forty-five women ranging in age from forty-two to eighty who were diagnosed with severe heart disease. The questionnaire consisted of five traditional female gender roles: wife/partner, mother, housekeeper, paid employee, and caregiver. For each role, participants were asked to rate their level of stress and satisfaction along a ten-point scale.

The women defined caregiving more broadly than the researchers did: rather than seeing it as a separate category, they felt it was part of all five roles. But they rated the roles differently. For example, they found being a wife equally satisfying and stressful; motherhood they found more satisfying than stressful; and caregiving, like marriage, got mixed reviews. On the one hand, women felt caregiving gave them a sense of purpose, meaning, and community connection. But they admitted it interfered with their own healthcare and considered it a barrier to managing their own heart problems. Because they were so busy taking care of others, many hesitated to ask for or get help for themselves.[5]

Perhaps the most startling statistic along these lines is this: According to the Huffington Post, a 2015 McKinsey study reported that women do *75 percent* of all caretaking in the *world*, caring for children, parents, or other family members.[6] In the United States alone, close to 44 percent (66,400,000) of women between the ages of thirty-five and sixty-four are caring for an older relative.[7] In many countries, women end up working 2.5 hours per day more than men doing unpaid work, such as caregiving and housekeeping.[8]

In a 2019 interview at the Essence Festival in New Orleans, Michelle Obama spoke about women's proclivity for putting others first:

We have a hard time putting ourselves on our own priority list, let alone at the top of it. And that's what happens when it comes to our health as women. We are so busy giving and doing for others that we almost feel guilty to take that time out for ourselves . . . We need to start having some conversations about this as women. . . . Why is it so hard for us as women to put ourselves first?

We're Stressed.

Stress is another reason women minimize their own healthcare. A report issued by the Cleveland Clinic Foundation suggests that women sometimes take on more than they can handle, find it harder than men to say no to other people's requests, and often feel guilty if we can't please everyone.[9] Dr. DiGiacomo suggests that's partly because as women, we're taught to keep our feelings hidden, particularly if they might be difficult or unpleasant for others.[10] Indeed, we've stood in second place for so long that we may not even notice we're standing there. As you'll see in the last chapter, women have been devalued throughout history—our bodies pathologized, our emotions suppressed, and our opportunities for independence and autonomy greatly curtailed.

We Worry about Our Families.

Dr. Senada Hajdarevic, a researcher in nursing science and public health at Umeå University in Sweden, and her colleagues conducted a study designed to test the differences between how men and women decide to seek medical care.

They interviewed fifteen men and fifteen women diagnosed with malignant melanoma. They found that the women were so concerned about disturbing their families that they delayed calling the doctor. They wanted to be absolutely sure they had a "real" issue.

In general, the men paid little attention to their bodies and only learned they had suspicious marks from their wives, siblings, and friends who happened to notice them. But as soon as the marks were pointed out, the men quickly sought medical advice. The few men who delayed getting help attributed their delay to work rather than family responsibilities.

The women paid more attention to their bodies than the men and noticed their marks much more quickly. But after that, they took longer than the men to seek help. At first, some tried to treat the marks themselves with various ointments they purchased over the counter. (Note: there are *no* effective OTC treatments for melanoma.) They told the researchers they were unsure what the marks were and wanted to watch them so they could be absolutely sure the marks were serious.

If recognized and treated very early, melanoma can usually be cured. If patients wait too long, the cancer can metastasize to other parts of the body, where it becomes far more difficult to treat and is often fatal.

According to the American Cancer Society, in 2021, over seven thousand people are expected to die from melanoma.

But they described how uncomfortable they felt taking time away from family responsibilities. And they made assumptions about the doctor's "busy schedule" and worried about making an appointment that might turn out to be unnecessary. While they thought their own health was important, they placed it behind the needs of their families, children, grandchildren—and even what they assumed were the needs of the doctor.[11]

Some women take this same approach even when they think they might be having a heart attack. In an admittedly small study, doctors Sheila Turris from the University of British Columbia and Joy Johnson from Simon Fraser University in Canada interviewed sixteen women who experienced heart attack symptoms when they were at home. They wanted to know how long it took the women to seek medical help, how they arrived at their decisions, and how they interpreted their symptoms.[12]

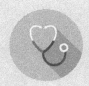 Heart attacks in women often present differently than they do in men. Because there is less common knowledge about this, many women delay going to the emergency room.

At first, the women were confused about what their symptoms meant. While some of them wondered if they were having a heart attack, others recognized that "something out of the ordinary was taking place in their bodies," but they couldn't put a name to it. They had some pain and felt dizzy, and normal tasks like taking a shower or cooking dinner became more difficult. But instead of calling the doctor, they tried to treat their symptoms themselves with nitroglycerine or over-the-counter antacids. Then they waited to see what, if anything, would happen.

They used some of the same excuses as the women in the melanoma study. They worried about feeling embarrassed, so they played down their symptoms and blamed them on stress or "dietary misadventures," even when other people who ate the same food felt just fine. When they finally realized they needed care, some still delayed asking for it. They worried about their work obligations and tried to be considerate of their family's schedule. One woman waited forty-eight hours before getting help, and another described staying awake all night and waiting until morning to go to the hospital because her partner worked fourteen-hour days and she felt he needed his rest. Many of the women ended up at the emergency room, and most of them went alone because they didn't want to upset their families and friends and subject them to potentially long waits.

Every forty seconds, an American will have a heart attack.

According to the Centers for Disease Control and Prevention, in 2019, heart disease caused one in every five female deaths in the United States. Over seven times more women died from heart disease than breast cancer (301,280 versus just under 42,000). The *University of California, Berkeley Wellness Letter* reported in 2012 that heart disease killed more women than all cancers, chronic respiratory disease, Alzheimer's, and accidents *combined*.[13]

This "watch and wait" trap is very familiar. I remember a couple of years ago I had what I thought was a stomach flu, which I typically get at least once a year. But this time, in addition to the usual vomiting and stomach cramps, I also began to perspire and feel clammy, symptoms I had never experienced before. I recall lying on the bathroom floor trying not to throw up and wondering whether it was my stomach or my heart.

I decided to watch and wait, figuring I would either get better or worse. Then the excuses sneaked up on me. I told myself it would be a shame to wake up my husband, scare him and my children to death, go to the hospital, complain about a possible heart attack, and then have my symptoms turn out to be nothing more than a bad case of stomach flu. What a waste of everyone's time!

As it happens, it *was* the stomach flu, and I got better very quickly. But my behavior wasn't all that different from the women in the melanoma and heart attack studies. What I didn't know until I researched this chapter was that my decision to watch and wait had the potential to kill me. It turns out that to minimize the damage from most heart attacks, the best thing you can do for yourself is to get treated within the first *four* hours.[14] So if you think you're having a heart attack, it's particularly dangerous to postpone getting help. After I told my doctor about the episode, he said, "Next time, call 911. When it comes to your heart, time equals muscle." And regardless of your symptoms, waiting to get help just isn't wise: waiting gives symptoms time to get worse and makes treatment and recovery more difficult.

When I talked with Melanie Johnson, for example, she said she wishes she'd worried less about her family and her work and more about herself. Several years ago, Melanie, a registered nurse, discovered a lump in her breast. Her nipples also looked different from usual, "like the skin of an orange," which she knew was a typical symptom of breast cancer. Since cancer runs in her family, she realized it was a real possibility:

> I knew I should check it out, but I was very involved with my work and my daughter. Then, after the original mammogram, they asked me to come back for a second test. But I didn't feel I had the time to go in right away. My husband was out of town, it was raining, work was really busy, and I didn't think I could find anyone who could take care of my daughter.

A couple of months later, she finally went for further testing and was diagnosed with Stage 3 invasive breast cancer. "I worried so much about my family and my job," she said, "that I didn't think about what breast cancer would mean for me and my life. As a result of my delay, I have a hard road ahead."

Remarkably, even after we've been told we need surgery, many women still choose to delay it rather than inconvenience the people around us. More women than men, for example, suffer from osteoarthritis, the most common form of arthritis. Women seem to have worse symptoms and more pain than men do, and we lose more cartilage and suffer greater disability. A common treatment for the condition is total joint arthroplasty (TJA), a surgical procedure in which parts of an arthritic or damaged joint are removed and replaced with a metal, plastic, or ceramic device called a prosthesis, which is designed to replicate the movement of a normal, healthy joint.

In 2011, Drs. Wendy Novicoff and Khaled Saleh, from the University of Virginia and Southern Illinois University Schools of Medicine, reviewed the TJA literature looking for differences between how men and women thought about TJA surgery. The first thing they found was that women are the majority of TJA patients. Then they noticed that both men and women seem to "underuse" the surgery, but that women are *three times* more hesitant to undergo it than men. In fact, some women complicated their recovery because they waited until the very last minute before finally consenting to have the operation. The researchers concluded that one reason for the women's delay was they didn't want to disrupt their role as family caregiver.[15]

Our caretaking mindset doesn't just stop us from calling the doctor. It also turns out that once we get our diagnoses, we often end up choosing treatments that fit most conveniently within our daily routines or those of our families.[16] While every patient needs to choose a treatment that makes sense with her time and resources, it's also important she select the one that's timely and best for her disease. As Melanie Johnson found out, selecting a treatment just because it fits most comfortably with our schedule or the schedule of the people around us can be dangerous and foolhardy.

Even more surprising is that although we frequently pick the treatments that we think will work best for everyone else, we still don't always follow through with them. It seems that women comply with treatment recommendations less often than men do partly because we prioritize our family or our work over our own needs—at the expense of our own health.[17]

Dr. Marie Manteuffel and her colleagues at the Centers for Medicare & Medicaid Services analyzed pharmacy and medical claims for 16 million adult women and 13.5 million men. During the analysis year, female patients filled more *new* drug prescriptions (not refills) than men (7.4 versus 6.2). But they found that women were *less likely* than the men to adhere to their medication regime, particularly for diabetes and cardiovascular medications. Approximately 12.6 million adult women have diabetes, but only 64 percent adhere to their recommended treatment. Sixty-four percent! That means that 36 percent, or 4.5 million women, failed to follow their doctor's treatment recommendations and likely won't reach their treatment goals.

What We Can Do About It

Michelle Obama had it right when she told Barbara Walters on the television show *20/20* that she makes herself her first priority. When asked if that could be seen as selfish, she said, "One of the things that I want to model for my girls is investing in themselves as much as they invest in others."

And I agree that's the first step in taking good care of our families. After all, if we're not in good shape, we can't take good care of others.

To help you *not* take a back seat when it comes to your own health, I've compiled a list of recommended preventative services for you to think about that will help keep you as healthy as possible. Of course, each of us needs to talk to our doctors and make our own decisions about which (or all) of these recommendations are appropriate. Your doctor may have other recommendations based on your age, insurance, and personal health profile.

❖ An annual checkup that includes blood pressure and weight monitoring, a cholesterol panel, a glucose test, an update on vaccinations, and whatever else the doctor recommends. Not everyone agrees on the necessity of annual exams. But I usually have one anyway since I like to keep tabs on what's happening in my body.

❖ Depending upon your risk factors, such as a family history of breast cancer, a clinical breast exam every year performed by your primary care doctor. If your risk factors are minimal, you may need it less frequently.

❖ A monthly breast self-exam. Here are a few things to look out for: changes in skin on your breast or nipple, including skin that looks like an orange peel; dimpling of the skin on the breast; any new hard, painless nodules on your breasts that do not change with your periods.

❖ A mammogram every year (I know that's open to debate).

❖ A bone mineral density test as needed, particularly after age sixty-five. And try to have a diet that is rich in calcium and vitamin D. Consider doing some resistance training as well.

❖ Starting around age fifty, a fecal screening test and/ or a colonoscopy, an exam used to detect changes or abnormalities in the large intestine (colon). A fecal screening test should be done yearly. If there is blood in your stool, the next step is a colonoscopy. Colonoscopies are done every ten years or as needed.

❖ A regular pelvic exam and pap smear to check for cervical cancer. Though I have them done annually, it's important to note that there is some disagreement about whether an annual pelvic exam is necessary. In fact, some doctors suggest getting one every three years unless abnormalities are noted. Talk with your doctor about whether he or she thinks it's important for you.

❖ A full body check from the dermatologist *at least* once a year to look for any unusual spots. And apply sunscreen when you go outside.

❖ An annual or biannual eye exam. And use sunglasses to protect your eyes when outside.

❖ A dental checkup and teeth cleaning, depending upon your needs, at least once or twice a year.

❖ An annual flu shot, or whatever shots your doctor suggests.

In addition to the above preventative services, remember to:

❖ Limit your alcohol. The Mayo Clinic suggests women limit their daily alcohol intake to twelve ounces of beer *or* one five-ounce glass of wine *or* 1.5 fluid ounces of 80-proof alcohol.
❖ Don't smoke.
❖ Try to get thirty minutes a day of exercise.

And whenever you're tempted to ignore any symptoms for a few days or hold off on calling the doctor because you just don't have time, remember the advice they give you every time you fly on a plane: put on your own oxygen mask *before* helping your children. As Michelle Obama says, all your good intentions toward others won't help you if you're not in good shape yourself.

CHAPTER 2

NICE GIRLS FINISH LAST

Our Reluctance to Question Our Doctor's Advice

For actress Rita Wilson, deciding to get a second opinion may well have saved her life. She told her story to *People* magazine and at the Huffington Post, where she is an editor at large. She explained, "I have had an underlying condition of LCIS (lobular carcinoma in situ), which is especially tough to diagnose and has been vigilantly monitored through yearly mammograms and breast MRIs."

She was relieved when two surgical breast biopsies showed no cancer. At some point, though, a friend convinced her to seek a second opinion, and the second pathologist found evidence of the disease. A third pathologist confirmed the finding of the second one, and, fortunately, Wilson was able to get effective treatment. She continues, "I am . . . expected to make a full recovery. Why? Because I caught this early, have excellent doctors, and because I got a second opinion."

In another interview with Health.com, Wilson explained why she decided to go public with her story: "I share this to educate others that a second opinion is critical for your health. You have nothing to lose if both opinions match up for the good, and everything to gain if something that was missed is found."

Unlike Wilson, many people don't get other opinions. The *Harvard Health Letter* reports that according to a poll conducted in 2010, 70 percent of all Americans don't bother to get second opinions—and, it turns out, that women are even less likely to get them than men are.[1] They can be critically important to us, however, since women are misdiagnosed more often than men, and we're prone to diseases that can be difficult for doctors to diagnose.[2]

 A Danish study found that across hundreds of diseases, women, on average, were diagnosed about four years later than men with the same disease: women received a cancer diagnosis 2.5 years after men; they received diagnoses for metabolic diseases, like diabetes, 4.5 years later.[3]

Why Women Hesitate to Get Second Opinions

Misdiagnoses can lead to a variety of problems, including death. There are several reasons for our general reluctance to question our doctor's advice.[4]

It's Not My Place.

We believe our doctors know best, so why should we question what they say? It can be uncomfortable to tell doctors that you're unsure about or disagree with their diagnosis. After all, they're the professionals.

It's Rude to Challenge the Doctor.

"If you don't have something nice to say, don't say anything at all." "You catch more flies with honey than vinegar." "Don't worry your pretty little head about it."[5] These are some of the cultural messages women receive and internalize, says Elisabeth Schuler Russell, President of the National Association of Healthcare Advocacy Consultants and founder of *Patient Navigator*, a blog designed to help patients become informed healthcare consumers. This socialization, she explains, can translate into a reluctance to question our doctors or get a second opinion.[6]

I Might Be Labeled a Difficult Patient.

One woman described her fear of this very real concern:

> I worry that if I ask for a second opinion, it implies that I mistrust my doctor's judgment and think he's incompetent. Worse, I'm afraid I might be considered a difficult patient. If a doctor notes that in my chart, that characterization could follow me from doctor to doctor like a permanent black mark.

There's a big difference, however, between badgering doctors, questioning everything they say, and being an informed consumer who wants to fully understand her situation. The problem, of course, is that no matter how thoughtfully and politely you ask your question, how you doctor interprets it is not within your control.

I Might Be Labeled Just Another "Hysterical Woman."

In 2006, Dr. Judith Lichtman, from the Yale School of Public Health, and some colleagues interviewed thirty women who had been hospitalized after a heart attack. She found that some of them were so afraid of being accused of "hysteria" that they had delayed calling the doctor.[7] This, too, is a credible concern. We *are* often labeled — if not hysterical, then overly emotional or prone to stress. Stacey Lewis received this diagnosis when she was a freshman in college.

She first realized something was wrong when she began inexplicably losing weight: "At first, it was just a pound or two, then five or six. My clothes stopped fitting, and I felt tired all the time."

She went to the campus health service and was told she was just homesick and stressed about college. It seems especially odd that they would jump to this conclusion, given that so many college students are prone to the exact opposite problem: the "freshman fifteen." She continued:

They focused on my weight loss and told me how many young college women struggle with body image. But my symptoms began to pile up. I developed purple bruises all over my body, painful periods, and an irregular heartbeat, but they stuck with their diagnosis. "Having lots of symptoms is common with anxiety and stress," they said.

Over the years, Stacey saw several other doctors who all arrived at a similar diagnosis. Even though none of them ever did a complete lab workup, she was given some unusual prescriptions, such as salt tablets, aloe juice, and glucose tablets to reduce her "stress." She said, "It felt like they were diagnosing me based on my age and gender, not my actual symptoms. They weren't listening, and I could tell they were labeling me just another hysterical woman. But I wasn't hysterical—I was sick!"

Finally, five years later, she saw a doctor who did the appropriate blood tests and found that she was suffering from Graves' disease, an autoimmune disorder that results in an overproduction of thyroid hormones. He did a procedure to address the problem, and she now takes a daily dose of Synthroid, a drug to help restore normal thyroid levels. For the first time in years, she says she feels great.

We Rush for Relief.

Second opinions take time and money, and some of the women I met felt too frightened and vulnerable to spend the time it would take to confirm their diagnosis and treatment options. Their aim was to move quickly to treatment in order to relieve their psychological and physical distress.

One woman told me, "A lot of women I know turn their authority over to their doctors the minute they get sick. That's because we all want help so badly that we become desperate. You just want to do it, whatever the 'it' is, and get it all over with."

That's what happened to me. I was so frightened I might be seriously ill that I plunged ahead with my surgery and put my brain on the back burner without thinking things through. In fact, it was a huge relief to defer to the doctor. Although I protested a little, it felt so easy to say finally, "Whatever you think, let's just do it now." In an emergency situation, of course, there's no choice. But when you're lucky enough to have the time, as I did, the desire to rush into treatment is not a useful attitude when you're trying to decide on the best course of action.

Misdiagnoses Are More Common Than We Think

In the *Journal of Evaluation in Clinical Practice*, Monica Van Such at the Mayo Foundation, and her colleagues, reported that of the 286 patients they looked at, 87 percent received a different or refined diagnosis with a second opinion.[8] Eighty-seven percent! That's *not* a typo!

And while we all know mistakes can happen, misdiagnosis is a serious issue. Twelve million Americans (men and women) are misdiagnosed each year, and women and minorities are 20 to 30 percent more likely to be misdiagnosed than [white] men.[9] One-third of those errors lead to serious disabilities or even death.[10] The recent COVID-19 crisis has changed this statistic, but, before COVID-19, *medical errors were the third leading cause of death* in the United States, right behind heart disease and cancer.[11]

Even when the consequences aren't so dire, a misdiagnosis can easily lead to patients getting the wrong treatment. A 2017 study by ProPublica, a nonprofit investigative journalism website, suggests it's common for patients to get treatments that research has shown are ineffective or even dangerous.[12]

Misdiagnoses happen for several reasons. One is that some doctors are just more competent than others. And some don't always keep up with the latest scientific information. That's understandable, since the scientific literature is so vast, and a doctor's time is so tight, but it's still cause for concern. Even if they do manage to keep up, what's shocking is that "newer" doesn't always mean "better." In 2013, a dozen doctors from around the country examined all 363 articles published in the *New England Journal of Medicine* over a decade, from 2001 to 2010, that tested a current clinical practice. Their

As I was writing this chapter, I received an email from a friend who is hard of hearing. She's getting older, and her hearing is deteriorating. She was advised by one doctor to get a cochlear implant, which involves surgically installing a small electronic device in the inner ear.

Cochlear implants are generally used only as a last resort for people with severe hearing loss who receive limited benefit from hearing aids. They don't work for everyone, and a real risk is that if they don't work, the surgery destroys any remaining hearing in the implanted ear.

What I found unbelievable was that no one had told her how problematic cochlear surgery can be. After we emailed a bit, she did some research, got a second opinion, and was advised *not* to do it. It turns out she's not even a candidate for it—her hearing isn't poor enough.

results found 146 studies that proved or strongly suggested that a current standard practice either had no benefit at all or was inferior to the practice it replaced. A different study conducted in 2012 by the Australian Department of Health and Ageing looked across the same decade and identified active medical practices that are probably either unsafe or ineffective.[13]

Why Misdiagnoses Occur

Misdiagnoses Happen for a Variety of Reasons. And some of them may surprise you.

Arriving at Accurate Diagnoses Can Be Difficult.

We may blame our misdiagnosis on negligence or incompetence. But that's not necessarily true. Arriving at a diagnosis can be difficult even in the best of circumstances, and, of course, any treatment we're recommended is based on our diagnosis. But figuring out what's wrong with someone is not a cut-and-dried process. In *Improving Medical Outcomes* (2011), a book about patient-doctor interaction, Dr. Fred Leavitt, professor of psychiatry at California State University, and attorney Jessica Leavitt explain some of the inherent complications:

> There are about twenty thousand known human diseases, many with several subtypes . . . a single disease may present itself in a dozen or more ways. In addition, there is considerable overlap among symptoms for various diseases.[14]

Medical schools know this, of course, which is why teaching students how to diagnose is uniquely difficult. Dr. Kathryn Montgomery, professor of medicine, medical humanities, and bioethics at the Northwestern University Feinberg School of Medicine in Chicago, describes the process:

> Medical students have traditionally been taught to do opposite things at once when they meet a new patient. They must suspend judgment, but form an initial impression; look for a single diagnosis to explain all symptoms, but watch for co-morbidities; avoid the anecdotal, but pay attention to stories; expect the diagnosis to be a common disease, but don't forget the rare ones.[15]

As I mentioned before, one reason women are often misdiagnosed is that we're prone to diseases that are difficult to diagnose. Autoimmune diseases, for example, affect more women than men and can take up to five years to diagnose correctly.[16] That's because many autoimmune diseases, such as lupus, rheumatoid arthritis, and Hashimoto's thyroiditis (an underactive thyroid gland), can have similar symptoms, which makes diagnosis more difficult because objective tests can't be as accurate. As a result, physicians may need to base their diagnosis on how the patient describes her symptoms and their own prior experiences of treating patients with similar symptoms—legitimate diagnostic tools, but not always the most accurate.[17]

And as Rita Wilson found out, even a breast cancer diagnosis is not a sure thing. Dr. Michael Sabel, a breast cancer surgeon at the University of Michigan, studied 149 breast cancer patients who, in one year alone, came to Michigan's Comprehensive Cancer Center after being diagnosed, biopsied, and given a treatment recommendation from another doctor elsewhere. They found that the specialty tumor board changed the treatments for *over half* of the women.

In one instance, for example, five patients were told to get a mastectomy when they were good candidates for breast-conserving lumpectomy instead. Other times, the original treatment advice didn't take into account newer techniques, such as using chemotherapy to shrink the tumor before operating so the breast could be saved. In 29 percent of patients, the pathologists at the specialty center interpreted biopsy results differently from the original doctors. Some women, for example, who were told their lump was not malignant did indeed have cancer.[18] While mistakes happen, that particular one can be a killer.

Gender Bias Can Be a Problem.

Sometimes, of course, misdiagnoses can be traced back to plain old gender bias. Women have been routinely omitted from clinical trials, and gender has been underemphasized in health research and treatment recommendations. What this means is that the medical community knows less about women's bodies than they do about men's and is therefore less likely to understand how a particular disease may manifest differently in women and men.[19]

Heart attacks, for example, are often missed in women—a mistake that can be fatal. A 2016 study from the University of Leeds in England looked at six hundred thousand heart attack patients over the course of nine years. It found that women have a 50 percent higher chance than men of receiving the wrong initial diagnosis following a heart attack. The researchers point out that the initial diagnosis is vital since it shapes treatment in the short run (and sometimes the long term as well). In fact, women (and men) who were misdiagnosed had approximately a 70 percent increased risk of death after thirty days compared with those whose diagnosis was accurate. They concluded that women's chances of misdiagnosis were so high because doctors typically expect a person with a heart attack to be an overweight, middle-aged man who has diabetes and smokes.[20] Obviously, that's not always the case.

Even before a heart attack actually occurs, unconscious gender bias can color a diagnosis of heart disease. Dr. Gabrielle Chiaramonte, a clinical psychologist at Weill Cornell Medical College, conducted a study in which internists and family physicians read a vignette of a forty-seven-year-old male or a fifty-six-year-old female at equal risk for heart disease. Each vignette presented the same variety of risk factors and heart disease symptoms, but half of them included sentences indicating that the patient had recently experienced a stressful event; the other half omitted any mention of stress at all. Each physician read one version of the vignette and diagnosed the patient based on the symptoms it described. When stress *wasn't* mentioned, there was no gender bias in the diagnoses. But when it was, only 15 percent of the women received a cardiac diagnosis compared to 56 percent of the men.[21]

A stress diagnosis can be particularly problematic because it feeds into a problem some women already tend to have, which is that we mistrust our symptoms to begin with and blame ourselves for just complaining. So if we're told our symptoms are due to stress, or something "just" psychological, we may be less likely to ask for a second opinion because it confirms what we thought in the first place: "I'm probably just a stress case, so why question the doctor?" Remember Stacey Lewis, whose initial misdiagnosis of stress kept her from learning for years that her real issue was Graves' disease?

Pain is another area where women don't fare so well. In "The Girl Who Cried Pain" (2001), a seminal study about women's experiences with the treatment of pain, Diane Hoffman, director of the Law and Health Care Program at the University of Maryland, and Dr. Anita Tarzian, also from the University of Maryland, concluded that doctors are less likely to take a woman's pain seriously than a man's — and more likely to characterize it as "emotional."[22] As a result, women are prescribed more sedatives and less pain medication than men are.

"The Girl Who Cried Pain" was published in 2001, and it's easy to think that things must have changed dramatically in twenty years. But in 2013, with *In the Kingdom of the Sick*, Laurie Edwards dispels that notion:

> Research shows that men who report pain are more likely to receive painkillers for their symptoms while women are given antidepressants and are more likely to have their pain dismissed as "emotional," "psychogenic," and "not real."[23]

Perceptual Bias Also Interferes.

And gender bias isn't the only kind of preconception that can color a doctor's diagnosis. There are also perceptual biases that can cause us to see what we *expect* to see. Dr. Jerome Groopman is professor of medicine at Harvard Medical School, chief of experimental medicine at Beth Israel Deaconess Medical Center, and one of the world's leading researchers in cancer and AIDS. In *How Doctors Think* (2007), he writes that while a competent doctor can rule out many diseases, a diagnosis can change depending upon the kind of doctor you go to: the exact same symptoms can suggest stomach problems to a gastroenterologist, muscle and joint issues to a rheumatologist, or stress to a psychologist.[24]

Perceptual bias may also cause patients to receive what I call an automatic or "generic" diagnosis just because they belong to a particular age, gender, racial, or any other group. That's what happened to my mother. When she was seventy, she went into the hospital as an outpatient to have knee surgery. Before the operation, she was totally sharp; there wasn't a senile bone in her body.

The surgery itself went fine, and she was sent home with instructions to take the prescribed pain pills twice a day. After a few days on the pills, she was confused and couldn't remember her name, address, phone number (except she remembered perfectly the phone number of her beauty shop!) or where she was. We took her back to the internist and, sure enough, she flunked all his memory tests. My father and I were positive her problems were due to the medication; the doctor insisted they weren't. I argued that she had been completely coherent before the surgery: no one becomes senile in a few days. The only change had been the medication. The doctor ignored what I said and asked to speak to me privately.

"I know it's hard," he told me gently. "But you're making your parents feel bad. They're aging, and you need to let them age gracefully."

I didn't say anything else, but I was furious. Why would my mother suddenly start aging so dramatically? Dad and I threw out the pills, and, sure enough, she recovered quickly. It turned out she was highly allergic to one or more of the ingredients that were in the medication, which is why her reaction had been so dramatic.

This particular doctor had been our internist for many years and was an excellent and caring physician. He knew how close our family was and how difficult it was for me to see my parents getting older. But because of my mother's age, he never looked for other reasons for her sudden confusion.

The bottom line is that women need second opinions to ensure their diagnosis is accurate, treatment isn't delayed, symptoms don't get worse, and the prescribed treatment is appropriate.

What We Can Do About It

You don't necessarily need a second opinion for every condition that sends you to the doctor. In an emergency situation, when time is of the essence, we need to follow through immediately with what our doctor suggests. And if you live in a more rural area with fewer resources, it may be logistically difficult to get a second opinion.

That said, there are some situations that almost always benefit from a second opinion. Yalemedicine.org recommends getting a second opinion for these five in particular:

❖ When the diagnosis is cancer
❖ When surgery is recommended
❖ When the diagnosis or treatment is unclear
❖ When the patient is your child
❖ When you want some peace of mind

A lot depends on whether the diagnosis *feels* right. If you disagree with or don't understand your doctor, if your questions aren't answered to your satisfaction, or if your diagnosis is ambiguous or potentially life-threatening, a second opinion is in order. You might also want one if your treatment requires surgery and/or drugs with serious side effects.

But before taking that extra step, *Consumer Reports on Health* suggests you ask the doctor the following questions about any diagnosis you receive.[25] If you feel perfectly satisfied with the answers, you may be fine without another opinion. However, to repeat what Rita Wilson said, if you decide to get a second opinion, "you have nothing to lose if

Patientadvocate.org suggests that you call your insurance provider before seeking any treatment or second opinion to prevent any confusion or denial of the bill. You need to know what they will cover—an out-of-network provider, any lab work or testing, and what your responsibilities are—before seeking a second opinion. Many insurance providers will not pay for second diagnostic tests if they were already completed for the initial diagnosis. You have the right to have copies of all tests you've had done.

Most insurance plans will pay for at least part of the cost of a second opinion. Medicare will pay 80 percent of the cost. If the second opinion disagrees with the first, Medicare will pay 80 percent of the cost of a third opinion. Patients who belong to an HMO are entitled to a second opinion, but some plans require a referral from your primary physician.

both opinions match up for the good, and everything to gain if something that was missed is found."

- ❖ What evidence supports this particular diagnosis and treatment recommendation?
- ❖ What other disease(s) could it possibly be?
- ❖ What are the benefits and risks of this particular treatment?
- ❖ What other treatment choices or alternatives do I have?
- ❖ What happens if I do nothing?

It can always be helpful to repeat, in your own words, what you heard the doctor say. Repeating what you've heard helps you avoid misunderstandings and ensure that you understood correctly.

If you decide you do want a second opinion, don't be afraid to ask your doctor for a recommendation. You might think she would be offended, but that's generally not the case. In fact, if your doctor *is* offended, that's not a good sign, and you might even want to look for someone else to serve as your primary physician.

You could also start by asking a family member or trusted friend for a recommendation. If possible, I suggest *not* going to another physician in the same office. The idea is to get a fresh approach from someone with different training and a different medical philosophy. If you're asking your family or friends, be sure to have them tell you about their experience with that person in some detail. Just because they like someone doesn't necessarily mean they're medically savvy.

It's also important to do some research on whomever you're considering. I was surprised to find how many people don't. In 2008, the American College of Surgeons conducted a nationwide survey and found that the average patient devotes an hour or less to researching his or her recommended surgery or surgeon. They also found that more than a third of patients who had an operation in the last five years never reviewed the credentials of their surgeon. Incredibly, patients are likely to spend way more time researching a new car (about eight hours) or a job change (about ten hours) than they are about the operation they're about to undergo or the surgeon who will perform it.[26]

Here are some issues to consider when researching any doctor:

❖ What are their credentials? When and where were they trained?

❖ Do they have any malpractice or sanctions listed?

❖ What hospitals are they associated with? What is the rating of their particular hospital on the procedure or surgery you're about to undergo?

❖ If you need surgery, how many times have they performed your particular operation? In other words, if you need a hip replacement, don't just go to an orthopedist. Find an orthopedist who does lots of hip replacements or, better yet, someone who specializes in them.

There's a lot of good information online, so if you have access to a computer, make use of it. But be careful. There's also a lot of misinformation out there. I try to avoid .com websites since they're less reliable than .edu or .gov sites. At the back of this book, I suggest websites that offer reliable information.

Once you decide whom to see, be sure take reports or actual images of any tests you've had to the second doctor. (Or ask to have them transferred electronically.) It's not unusual for different radiologists to read the same image differently or for different pathologists to have a different take on the same biopsy.[27]

What to Do with a Second Opinion

If time is not an issue, it's best to give yourself enough time to mull over what you've heard. The mere passage of time tends to put things in a different perspective. Talk to anyone you can find who has experienced what you are going through, and check to see if there are support groups of people who have your disease and can share their experiences.

Then, take what you've learned back to your original doctor so you can discuss it and put it all in perspective. I've found most doctors very helpful in addressing my concerns. But if you find your doctor resists answering your questions, or if you can't reconcile the conflicting approaches, you may need to seek an additional opinion. Hopefully, by then, some consensus will emerge.

I suggest taking a trusted person with you to your appointment to ensure you don't miss any information that's discussed. And be sure to take notes during your visit and clarify anything you don't understand.

In a worst-case scenario, you can get caught in an internecine war, which will really complicate your decision-making. In the 1980s, when our eldest daughter, Lisa, was eighteen, she developed TMJ (temporomandibular joint disorder), a jaw disorder in which chewing becomes quite painful. The condition is more common in women than in men.[28] The jaw is a ball-and-socket joint, similar to our hips, with a disc of cartilage that rides between the two joints. In Lisa's case, her disc had slipped, and her bones were making direct contact. Each time she chewed, it was bone against bone.

At the time, one of the recommended treatments was a discectomy, or disc removal, in which a surgeon removes the original disc and replaces it with a Teflon disc. However, that treatment carried a major risk: it was possible that during the surgery, one or more of the facial nerves could be nicked, which can cause partial paralysis of the face. Since the potential ramifications were so terrifying, we decided to find out if there were other options.

Fortunately, we lived in Los Angeles, where there were plenty of professional resources. We were also fortunate that we had the financial resources, since our insurance at the time wouldn't cover us. My husband and I took Lisa to many different specialists—dentists, orthodontists, periodontists, and oral surgeons—but they disagreed with each other about what to do.

It turned out there were two camps in the TMJ community: one was 100 percent for surgery; the other, 100 percent against it. There seemed to be no middle ground. An expert in the surgery camp went so far as to say, "If you don't allow your daughter to have the surgery, I strongly suggest *you* get psychological therapy. You really need to think about your unconscious hostility toward your daughter."

I tried to weigh that against the expert in the let-it-be camp who said, "If it were my daughter, I would just wait and see. Mothers who rush their children into inappropriate treatments need to examine their motives. Our children don't need to be perfect."

I felt completely put down by both comments. Even though my husband was present at all of the appointments, those comments were directed solely toward me. I was labeled a neurotic mother. As you can imagine, since we found none of those doctors to be particularly appealing, my husband, daughter, and I decided to figure out what to do by ourselves. After much discussion, we all concluded that since delaying the surgery wouldn't be fatal, we should put it off. Our thinking was that she could always go back and have it later if chewing became too painful and interfered with her quality of life. By that time, we figured, newer techniques with fewer side effects might be available. Fortunately, her TMJ has settled into a manageable state, and now, while her jaw isn't perfect, it only occasionally hurts.

For years we all wondered whether or not we did the right thing in letting it go. It was only later that we felt vindicated: It turned out that the Teflon implant caused a severe reaction associated with bone destruction, pain, and even severe facial disfigurement. As a result, it has been withdrawn from the market.

Sometimes an ounce of caution is all it takes to avoid being one of the twelve million outpatient Americans who are misdiagnosed each year or who receive a less effective or even the wrong treatment.[29]

CHAPTER 3

TURNING INWARD

Blaming Ourselves for Getting Sick

Margaret Adams, sixty-two, lives in a small town in Texas. She's an artist, and she owned her own retail business for over twenty years. Margaret suffers from Sjögren's disease, an autoimmune system disorder that can affect multiple parts of the body. Sjögren's often causes dry eyes and dry mouth to the point where your eyes feel as if they're full of sand and your mouth feels as if it's stuffed with cotton. It can be difficult to swallow or talk. It can also be associated with joint pain, profound fatigue, neuropathy, and cognitive impairment, and it can affect major organs.

An estimated one to four million Americans have Sjögren's syndrome. The disease affects people of all races, ethnicities, and ages. However, women are nine times more likely to develop this condition than men.[1]

Margaret is positive she caused her Sjögren's disease:

At the time of my Sjögren's diagnosis, I was trying to sell my business and, at the same time, I was
forced to move, since they were tearing the building
down. I moved to a terrible neighborhood that was
the only one I could afford. What a big mistake! But
despite not feeling well, I had to go in and work and
try to save what I could.

I'm sure my phenomenal stress caused my Sjögren's.
The stress of moving my business and becoming ill, it's
all wrapped up in my mind with the feeling of failure
over the business collapsing a couple of years later. So
then it becomes a big self-blame issue.

As a group, women tend to blame themselves easily and
often. The women I met were consistently ashamed of being
ill and believed their illness reflected their inability to properly
manage their lives. I talked with women who suffered from a
variety of diseases—lupus, endometriosis, breast cancer, and
rheumatoid arthritis, to name just a few. While their reasons
for blaming themselves were personal and individual, shame
was their common denominator.

When Beth Tiner (Beth asked me to use her real name),
for example, was in college, she began having extremely painful menstrual cycles. She told me, "When I got my period,
it felt like I had swallowed a live piranha. It was eating me
from the inside out. I knew my cramps were worse than
everyone else's, but at first, it never occurred to me to call
the doctor."

Beth was attending a conservative religious university that she loathed and was trying desperately to adjust. Then her grandmother, with whom she was extremely close, died from cancer. "I was so homesick and lonely," she said. "That's why I assumed my stress was causing my terrible cramps. It was all just too much for me to handle."

Not only did Beth blame herself for bringing on her cramps; she was equally hard on herself for what she thought was her inability to tolerate them: "I kept trying to suck it up and tough it out. Everyone has stress, and all women have cramps. Why was I whining so much?"

When Beth returned home during Easter break, she went immediately to the doctor, who diagnosed endometriosis, a painful disorder in which tissue that normally lines the inside of the uterus—the endometrium—grows outside it. During menstruation, the displaced tissue gets trapped and can't be sloughed off the way normal endometrial tissue is. That's why it hurts so much.

She tried a number of pain medications, but nothing worked. Finally, she had a hysterectomy, a treatment of last resort for endometriosis. Unfortunately, she had a tougher time recovering from surgery than she expected. Her energy was low, her bones ached, and she was on multiple medications for thyroid issues, migraine headaches, and insomnia. And, as she put it, "My sexual desire went down the toilet."

Beth did some research and knew that after hysterectomies other women experience similar symptoms. In fact, her exact symptoms are commonly reported. According to the Danish Pain Research Center, pain is present in 17 to 32 percent of women after a hysterectomy.[2] The *International Journal of Surgery* reported that hysterectomies also increase the prevalence of migraines, and the journal *Current Sexual Health Reports* suggests that after a hysterectomy, approximately 20 percent of women suffer from diminished sexual function.[3]

According to the *New York Times*, women who have a hysterectomy have an increased risk of depression and anxiety.[4]

Nevertheless, she was still ashamed that she recovered so slowly and was unable to shake the belief that she was "more whiny than most." "Everyone has hysterectomies," she said. "Why couldn't I just get over it like everyone else? What's the matter with me?"

Extensive research provides example after example of how prevalent guilt and shame are among women.[5] It's important to note, however, that shame and guilt are two different feelings. Shame, especially, eats away at our sense of self. In a TED Talk, Dr. Brené Brown, a research professor at the University of Houston, said that Jungian analysts call shame the "swampland of the soul." She explains:

Shame is a focus on self; guilt, a focus on behavior.

Guilt says, "I *did* something bad. I'm sorry. I made a mistake."

Shame says, "I *am* bad. I'm not good enough. I'm sorry. I'm a mistake."

For example, one woman I met said to me, "It's my own fault I got sick. I've had so much going on at work, I just haven't had time to take good care of myself lately." That's guilt.

Others internalized the blame, saw their illness as reflecting and confirming their inability to live, what one woman called "a disciplined life." She said to me, "I never take care of myself. I rarely exercise; I shouldn't smoke. I'm a hot mess. No wonder I got sick!" That's shame.

Self-blame is such a deep trap that even death and grief can't escape it. It's truly amazing to realize how hard on ourselves some of us can be even when few—if any—people would blame us for feeling the way we do.

I originally contacted Dr. Robbie Davis-Floyd, an adjunct professor in the Department of Anthropology at Rice University in Houston, to see if she had done any research on the subject of women and self-blame. To my surprise, she asked to participate in my research as a case study.

In 2000, Robbie's only daughter, Peyton, was killed in an automobile accident while driving home to celebrate her twenty-first birthday. The driver was Peyton's nineteen-year-old friend, who glanced away from the road to change a CD. Realizing she'd drifted off the road, she swung the steering wheel so hard to get back on it that the car flipped four times, sending Peyton through the windshield and fifty feet down the highway. Even with such an unimaginable tragedy, Robbie still blames herself for not doing better in dealing with her daughter's death:

About a year after Peyton's death, I woke up one morning and found I couldn't get out of bed. My world just collapsed. I had run out of strength, energy, and willpower, and I began to have an enormous number of physical and emotional problems. How could I let myself fall into a depression? I believed that strong people like I had been before Peyton's death should be strong enough to just choose to rise above it. My family and friends thought I just needed to develop some self-discipline. Never mind that I had an enormous amount of self-discipline before my daughter's death. I knew better, but I felt like a lazy, guilty, irresponsible jerk.

Nine years later, when I met Robbie, she still felt pretty much the same. Despite all of her degrees and the amount of time that had passed since Peyton's death, she couldn't let up on herself and see her symptoms as a perfectly logical response to her devastating loss. Her family's motto of "Rise above it" had sunk in too deeply, and shame became her default position. She wanted to share her story to let women know they're not alone in feeling shame—that regardless of their particular experience, level of education, or number of credentials, self-blame can be irrational and tenacious.

In a study conducted between 1996 and 1998, Rosemary King from the University of Ballarat in Victoria, Australia, interviewed twelve men and twelve women with a provisional diagnosis of a heart attack. Seventeen of the twenty-four participants blamed their illness on stress. The men externalized their stress—they considered work the main cause of their problems—while the women internalized it, describing themselves as "prone to worry." They assumed it was their particular personality trait that caused their illness.[6]

Dr. Donna Stewart at the University of Toronto similarly found that out of the four hundred breast cancer survivors she studied, more women blamed their condition on stress than genetics, hormones, diet, or any other factor.[7] And in 2007, Dr. Lois Friedman, a professor of psychiatry at Case Western Reserve University in Cleveland, and her colleagues found that more than half of the 123 breast cancer patients they surveyed believed their disease occurred because they had difficulty coping with stress and because they were anxious, nervous, and overly pessimistic.[8]

But our "inability" to handle stress isn't the only thing that we believe makes us sick. As a group, women are amazingly good at finding all sorts of reasons to blame ourselves and feel ashamed. When Desireé Daruma was diagnosed with lupus, she did a lot of research and discovered that lupus is a serious disease that can affect major organs. Its symptoms may include joint pain, headaches, confusion, memory loss and fatigue. For Desireé, fatigue was the most debilitating:

> I never knew what tired was until I got lupus. I can't even use the word *fatigue*. There were days I was so exhausted that I couldn't even lift my arms to brush my teeth. I gauged how well I was doing by whether I could get up and make the bed. To me, that was already a good day.

While women are less susceptible to infections than men are, autoimmune diseases affect more of us than men. Approximately five million people suffer from lupus worldwide, and nine out of ten of them are women.[9]

Desireé understood that the cause of lupus remains unknown, but, despite all her research, she still firmly believed that, in her case, her childhood behavior was to blame. She described herself as a fat child who was disliked and teased by the girls at school. To retaliate, she became a bully and beat up some of them so badly that a few required stitches. "Everything has a meaning or a purpose," she told me. "I'm sure my illnesses are total payback for the people I've hurt during my life."

Sadly, the tendency to view illness as punishment for past behavior is common. In 1994, Dr. Elizabeth Klonoff, from California State University, and Dr. Hope Landrine, from East Carolina University, interviewed 178 undergraduate students (56 men and 122 women) about their thoughts on the causes of illness. The researchers compiled a list of six diseases: headache, high blood pressure, AIDS, the common cold, diabetes, and lung cancer. Then they provided a list of potential causes, including emotional distress, punishment for wrongdoing, sin, anger and anxiety, genes/heredity, and germs/infection, among others, and they asked the men and women to attribute a cause to each disease. While both men and women said that AIDS was punishment for sin or sexual activity, the women were more likely than the men to view other illnesses that way as well.[10]

Of course, it's important to remember that sometimes we *can* be partly responsible for causing our illness. We may smoke even though we know it can cause lung cancer, or we may drink excessively even though we know it's a risk factor for breast cancer and can cause cirrhosis of the liver.

constitute a risk to health in themselves but reflect the individual's ability to have regular screening and to take preventative action. Equally, risks to over-eating and overweight are seen in terms of self-control, the breakdown of restraint . . . the individual has become at risk from his or herself.[13]

All that focus on individual responsibility isn't fair because we know (or *should* know) that randomness—and genetics—also play a huge role in one's health. That's why we can do all the right things and still become ill; we can do all the wrong ones and still remain healthy. My father-in-law, for example, smoked cigars daily, loathed vegetables, loved red meat, rarely exercised, and never got sick until the day he died at eighty-four. I, on the other hand, do all the "right things," and my blood pressure is a lot higher than his ever was. You just never know.

Even before the wellness movement, there was Dr. Norman Vincent Peale's hugely popular dictum on the power of positive thinking: he maintained that the key to good health and wellness was to stay positive and think cheerful, optimistic thoughts.

In *Bright-Sided: How the Relentless Promotion of Positive Thinking Has Undermined America* (2009), Dr. Barbara Ehrenreich, who has a PhD in cell biology, discovered these expectations during her own experience with breast cancer: "There was, I learned, an urgent medical reason to embrace cancer with a smile: a 'positive attitude' is supposedly essential to recovery . . . it remains almost axiomatic within the breast cancer culture that survival hinges on 'attitude.'"[14]

Indeed, in 2000, Dr. Donna Stewart and colleagues surveyed two hundred women in Canada and the United States whose ovarian cancer was in remission and found that over 82 percent felt that their disease failed to recur because they maintained a "positive attitude."

It makes sense that a positive attitude is a good thing. You certainly won't find many people arguing that it's better to be miserable and depressed when dealing with illness. But the fact is, the scientific jury is still out on how much of a connection there really is between mental outlook and physical health. In *Bright-Sided*, Dr. Ehrenreich writes about Dr. Ilona Boniwell, a professor of positive psychology in England, who suggests that the *science* of positive psychology has not necessarily caught up with its *promise*.[15]

And in fact, some research suggests that trying to feel happy in the face of illness is *not* necessarily healthy. It can make us reluctant to admit the severity of our disease and slower to seek treatment and to follow through on recovery strategies.

The Guardian, a newspaper published in Great Britain, reported that Macmillan Cancer Support, a large British charity that provides information, care, and financial support to people affected by cancer, said its research showed that one of the biggest barriers to honest conversations about dying was the pressure to stay positive, even when patients received a terminal diagnosis. Pressure to see themselves as a "fighter," "battling" against cancer, can help some people remain upbeat about their disease; for others, however, the effort of keeping up a brave face is exhausting and unhelpful in the long term.[16]

Self-Blame Has Consequences

Although it may seem counterintuitive, blaming oneself for becoming ill can actually be helpful to some people. Dr. Rita Charon, director of the program in narrative medicine at the Columbia University College of Physicians and Surgeons, explains that self-blame can help answer the question we all ask when we become ill: "Why me?" She says:

> Illness seems to induce irrational guilt in patients who search for *something* they may have done to cause their lymphoma or breast cancer or multiple sclerosis. Identifying something concrete in their experience that caused their illness seems preferable to accepting its random unfairness, even at the cost of assuming some of the responsibility for their illness themselves.[17]

As Dr. Charon points out, blaming ourselves when we feel frightened or vulnerable makes some sense. The sense of control it offers can be helpful when we have to face a scary diagnosis. However, Dr. Jill Kane, a psychologist in Northern California, says the problem with this approach is that the control we think we have isn't real:

> We say to ourselves, "If it's my fault, then maybe I can do something about it." That implies I have the power to make my issues disappear, which may or may not be a true assessment. "Real control" is taking responsibility for those things we actually *can*

control, such as following up with our medical care, getting that second opinion, and complying with our treatment regimen. It's letting go of things we can't do anything about, like genetics, past behavior, or just plain randomness.

It's pretty clear that, in most cases, the drawbacks of self-blame outweigh its benefits. Women may feel so embarrassed and ashamed about getting sick that they delay calling the doctor, a lapse that can sometimes turn a minor problem into a major—or even fatal—one.

In 1998 and 1999, Dr. Helen Richards and her colleagues interviewed sixty men and women between the ages of forty-five and sixty-four in Glasgow, Scotland, who were experiencing chest pain. After family history, most of the participants blamed their health problems on their own behavior. Because they felt their doctors would blame them as well, many of them hesitated to make that call. Some even believed that because they had "caused" their disease, their health problems deserved lower priority than those of other people who might "really be sick."[18]

So the repercussions from self-blame are very real and place a kind of double burden on us. Not only do we have to devote time and energy to getting better, we also have to deal with the added guilt and shame that come from thinking it's all our own fault.

What We Can Do About It

When I began this chapter, I had hoped to write that if you're a woman who blames herself for becoming ill, here are six or seven or eight steps you can take to make the blame disappear. Unfortunately, it's not that simple. As I've discussed, the reasons why we blame ourselves are personal and complex, most likely a mix of our genetics, our upbringing, and our cultural environment.

Yet, while there are no easy answers or quick fixes, there are coping strategies that can help us deal with self-blame and the shame and guilt it can cause.

Acknowledging that you're blaming yourself is the first step, and I think it's the most important. Many of the feelings that lead women to blame themselves are so deeply ingrained that we're unaware we have them. And you can't resolve an issue if you don't even know it exists.

Another of the most helpful things to do is to join a support group of women dealing with similar problems. Sharing your feelings with a group and realizing you're not alone can itself be hugely therapeutic. Plus, learning how other women deal with self-blame can give you ideas for your own journey.

If you can afford it, therapy or counseling can also be useful. And there's research to suggest that journaling, or writing about our experiences—both positive and negative ones—can help people deal better with them.

In 2004, Drs. Chad Burton from the University of Pittsburgh and Laura King from the University of Missouri selected ninety undergraduates, twenty-four men and sixty-six women. They divided them into two groups and asked each group to write for twenty minutes on three consecutive days. Group One was instructed to write about one of the most wonderful experiences in their lives. Group Two was told to write about a neutral topic, such as "In as much detail as possible, write about your plans for the rest of the day" or "Write a description of the shoes you are wearing."

The students who wrote about their positive experiences reported significantly fewer visits to a health center for the next three months than the neutral group. And it wasn't just about getting to a doctor; the first group also remained healthier.[19]

What I found particularly fascinating is that in a previous study, Dr. Joshua Smyth and his colleagues achieved the same results using the *opposite* approach. They selected fifty-eight asthma patients and forty-nine patients with rheumatoid arthritis and also divided them into two groups: Group One was asked to write for twenty minutes on three consecutive days about the most stressful event in their lives. Patients wrote about the death of a loved one, serious relationship issues, or having experienced a major disaster, such as a train wreck. Group Two wrote about neutral experiences along the lines of the Burton and King study. It turned out that 47 percent of the patients who wrote about their negative thoughts showed improvement, compared to only 24 percent of the control group.[20]

The obvious conclusion seems to be that just writing about life is a viable coping strategy. Dr. James Pennebaker, a social psychologist, suggests that making a story out of a messy complicated experience can make the experience more graspable. It gives us the opportunity to stand back and evaluate where we are in life so we can perhaps change our perspective.[21]

At the back of this book, I've included several websites that can help women navigate these difficult issues.

Remember, the tendency to blame ourselves can be a difficult, if not impossible, habit to break; it may be necessary to try a variety of techniques in order to find the most helpful ones. But it's definitely worth doing. Removing or at least diminishing the burdens of guilt and shame may or may not relieve our symptoms, but doing so can help us call the doctors more quickly, make us less hesitant to ask questions, and make us more diligent about seeking second opinions. Guilt and shame are bitter pills to swallow, and they're not the ones we need when adjusting to or recovering from illness.

CHAPTER 4

MEDICAL CROSSTALK

"What We Have Is a Failure to Communicate"

"The single biggest problem in communication is the illusion that it has taken place."
—George Bernard Shaw

As Deborah Richards, forty-two, quickly discovered, doctors and patients can have vastly different points of view.

A high-powered attorney, Deborah works over sixty hours a week for a large law firm, where she hopes to become a partner. Deborah has always been healthy, but she worries about her potentially high risk for breast cancer. She's an Ashkenazi Jew,[1] she never had children (according to breastcancernow.org, women who have given birth have a lower *lifetime* risk for breast cancer), and her grandmother had breast cancer in her early fifties. Because of all this, her doctor had urged her numerous times to have a BRCA blood test to determine whether she has a genetic predisposition for developing the disease. BRCA1 and BRCA2 are human genes that produce tumor-suppressor proteins. When these genes are altered (mutated), the tumor-suppressor proteins are no longer functional, which can lead to cancer. The blood test detects mutations in those genes, and women with the mutation have a much higher risk for developing breast cancer.

Deborah remained adamant that she didn't want to take the test, and when we met, she and her doctor had reached a stalemate. She told me, "Because my risk is so high, my doctor told me that if the test turned out positive, I would have several options: on the radical side, I could have a double mastectomy, just in case. Or I could take some serious medications, some of which have severe side effects, to try and prevent the cancer from happening. Or I could just do nothing, continue my yearly mammograms, and wait on pins and needles to see if cancer developed."

Deborah found all of those choices terrible. She continued, "Obviously, I was really worried about someday developing cancer. And if that time came, I would make the decisions I need to make. But a positive result would have made me feel like a ticking time bomb. My anxiety would have been overwhelming."

Several years later, Deborah finally decided to have the test because she realized she was worried and anxious anyway. She figured knowing her risks one way or the other might help. If the test proved negative, she could stop worrying; if it proved positive, at least she'd know for sure what she might be facing. Fortunately, the results proved negative, but she now thinks her doctor was right; she should have had the test when he first suggested it. Despite the anxiety the results might have caused, she feels that it's information every woman at risk needs to know.

But she added, "At the time it was really hard for me. My doctor just didn't get it."

Deborah and her doctor were at cross-purposes, the fault of neither but to the detriment of both. Doctors tend to have a narrower focus: on viruses, bacteria, biopsies, lab results, and worst-case scenarios. Patients worry about broader things: symptoms, anxieties, families, and jobs. Deborah's doctor failed to fully understand that at the time, Deborah just wasn't ready for a positive result, so it didn't make sense to push her to take the test.

My own experience was somewhat similar to Deborah's. I was sure my new hormone medications were causing my bleeding; my doctor was sure they weren't. He could have backed off and given me permission to revert to my old medication and wait a week or two to see whether my bleeding stopped. Instead, he pushed his own agenda and, at the same time, pushed mine aside. I know he was concerned for me. But even if he had been right and I did have some form of cancer, I doubt I would have keeled over in those two weeks. But my fright (and his) overtook what could have been a mutual dialogue of give and take.

A 2002 study confirmed that Deborah and I are not alone in feeling that our doctors didn't fully understand us. Dr. Richard Street, chief of the Health Decision-Making & Communication Program at the VA Medical Center in Texas, and Dr. Paul Haidet, from Penn State Hershey Medical Center, wanted to learn how well doctors understand what patients think about their illness.[2] They recruited twenty-nine physicians from the Veterans Administration, private practices, and public community-based clinics, plus 207 patients with a range of complaints, 39 percent of whom were women. After each patient-doctor visit, physicians and patients completed a testing instrument that measured the difference between what doctors thought their patients believed about their illness and what patients actually believed.

The differences, it turned out, were huge. Doctors believed patients thought their health issues had a biological cause, assumed patients understood how little control they had over them, and misjudged the amount of information patients wanted. But the patients didn't think like that at all. Because patients tend to see their illness as their fault, they minimized any biological basis for their disease and felt they had more control than the doctors assumed. Patients also wanted more information and to be more involved in choosing their treatment than the doctors realized.

There are some sound historical reasons behind doctors' tendency to underestimate the degree of involvement patients want, and in fact there were periods in history when a collaborative relationship between doctors and patients, the idea of them talking to one another, was actually frowned upon. Some doctors simply thought that the less patients understood, the more respect they would have for them and for science. In 1924, Dr. Daniel Cathell (1839–1925) advised young doctors to blind the patient with scientific jargon:

Working with the microscope and making analyses of the urine, sputum, blood, and other fluids as an aid to diagnosis will not only bring fees and lead to valuable information regarding your patient's condition, but will also give you reputation and professional respect, by investing you, in the eyes of the public, with the benefits of being a very scientific man. . . . By employing the terms ac. phenicum for carbolic acid, secale cornutum for ergot . . . you will debar the patient from reading your prescriptions.[3]

Why Clear Communication Is So Important

Things have changed since then—imagine how well that attitude would go over today—and, of course, most doctors certainly don't feel that way. Today, in fact, clear conversation is equally important to doctors and patients. In "Hurting All Over," an article he wrote for *The New Yorker*, Dr. Jerome Groopman says, "Language is as vital to the physician as the stethoscope or the scalpel."[4] That's because it turns out that more than 75 percent of the time, the key to a diagnosis comes from the patient's story.[5] For doctors, language helps them gain a clearer understanding of how we see our illnesses; for patients, particularly patients that suffer from illnesses for which there are no clear objective tests, our personal details might help doctors arrive at a more accurate diagnosis.

Dr. Howard Brody, director of the Center for Ethics & Humanities in the Life Sciences at Michigan State University, explains how all the technical aspects of care—physical exams, lab tests, and even a rigorously followed course of treatment—do not necessarily make patients feel better. Dr. Brody believes that good communication is the single most important secret to feeling better. By "good communication" he means whether or not patients feel they've had a chance to fully discuss their problem with their doctor and whether they think their doctor sees their problem the way they do."[6] Only after patients feel they have been listened to will they recognize the doctor's explanation as being about their own illness rather than just a quick, glib diagnosis.

When making a health care decision, a recent survey of ten thousand American patients found that 85 percent of Americans feel that a doctor's compassion is more important than cost.[7]

Research has confirmed Brody's ideas. In 2007, Richard Frankel, a professor of medicine at Indiana University School of Medicine, and his colleagues conducted a review of thirty-six studies and found that good doctor-patient communication made a measurable difference in how patients felt: it helped relieve some physical symptoms such as chronic headaches, it lowered blood sugar in diabetics, and it improved blood pressure readings in patients with hypertension.[8]

And a study from Massachusetts General Hospital in 2014 also found that a good doctor-patient relationship improved diagnoses. Patients who had good relationships with their doctors told them about symptoms they might otherwise not have disclosed and were also more likely to believe in and comply with their treatments, which, of course, increased the treatments' chances of success.[9]

But a good relationship with our doctors is not always easy to achieve. Other studies have found that often doctors do much of the talking and that they ask patients whether they understand what was discussed during their appointment only 1.5 percent of the time.[10] As women, we're socialized to take our turn in a conversation and to be friendly at all times. As a result, we don't always get to state all of our concerns. And, as these studies reveal, unless patients feel comfortable enough in the relationship to disclose their symptoms and ask for clarification, they may fail to understand and adhere to their treatment recommendations, which means that their recovery may be much more difficult.[11]

Women's Conversational Styles Can Interfere with Their Diagnoses

Women and men talk to doctors differently. Research has found that, as a group, women have some unique conversational styles that can get in the way of an accurate diagnosis.

We Describe Our Feelings.

In a seminal essay published in 1999 titled "Differences in Clinical Communication by Gender," Dr. Virginia Elderkin-Thompson, a neuropsychologist who specialized in researching brain disorders at UCLA, and Dr. Howard Waitzkin, a professor of sociology and a physician at the University of New Mexico, found that when women described their symptoms, they presented more complaints than men and spent more time describing their emotions: how they *felt* about being sick and about the stress it put them under and how worried they were about their families.[12] The men tended to be more succinct, objective, and reserved. They didn't want to "act like a baby," and they tried to keep "a stiff upper lip."[13]

Male and female doctors also have different conversation styles.

Female doctors spend about 10 percent more time with patients than male doctors and talk with them more. Female doctors communicate more positively, verbally and nonverbally, and are more emotionally responsive. They express empathy and concern more often and are more likely to ask about and provide counseling in the areas of lifestyle and mental health.

But when the conversation has a more biomedical focus, when it gets around to diagnosis, prognosis, and medical treatment, the differences disappear, and doctors' conversation styles are more similar.[14]

In 2008, Dr. Clive Seale, professor of sociology at Brunel University in the United Kingdom, and Dr. Jonathan Charteris-Black, from the Bristol Centre for Linguistics, arrived at similar results. They interviewed 102 cancer patients and purchased an additional 1,035 interview transcripts for a secondary analysis. They found that the older men in the study used words associated with gathering information and evidence and saw their illness as a technical problem to be solved. The older women used words that were more emotional, and they were more focused on sharing their experience with others. The language of the younger men and women was more similar, although some of those same differences still existed.[15]

In 2013, Laurie Edwards discussed how differently men and women described their pain. Women are vague and abstract while men use simple, concrete terms. Men simply report what hurts and where. In "The Girl Who Cried Pain," the authors say that women talk about their pain within the context of their relationships and social networks.[16]

Men and women's conversation styles are so different that patient gender can be identified just by reading letters. One hundred thirty medical and psychology students read eighty-one letters patients wrote about having cancer. Their task was to figure out which letters were written by men, which by women.

Students identified the patient's gender in 62 percent of the cases. Men's letters were shorter, used more formal language, and focused on facts. Many of the women's letters were longer, used language more vividly, and mentioned emotions and interpersonal relationships more often.[17]

These different speech patterns can have dire results. Dr. Gabrielle Chiaramonte offers this disturbing example:

> Considering gender differences in symptom presentation . . . the likelihood that women with CHD [congestive or end-stage heart disease] will also discuss life stressors and report symptoms of anxiety is high. . . . The likelihood that health care providers will be *influenced by the interaction of psychological symptoms and the patient's female gender is also*

high [italics mine]. . . . The incorrect assessment of symptom origin could therefore delay medical care in women with CHD.[18]

They can also lead to different diagnoses, even when the symptoms described are exactly the same. In 1993, Dr. Brian Birdwell from the University of Oklahoma Health Sciences Center and his colleagues selected forty-four internists, four of them women, and divided them into three groups. In a scripted patient-physician interview, two of the groups watched a video-tape of an actress performing the role of a patient with chest pain. The third group read the transcript but didn't watch the interview. The dialogue in the two videos and the transcript was identical, and all the groups had the same laboratory data and description of symptoms that pointed toward a cardiac diagnosis.

Group one saw the actress/patient describe her symptoms in a businesslike manner. She dressed conservatively, was unemotional, and stuck to the facts. Group two saw the same actress relate the same symptoms in exactly the same words, but this time she was dressed more brightly and wore a lot of jewelry. She was a lot more emotional, she used a lot more hand gestures, and she raised and lowered her voice more expressively.

Then the doctors were asked, "What is this patient's most likely diagnosis?" Doctors from the first group diagnosed cardiac issues, and all but one of them chose to pursue a noninvasive cardiac workup for the patient.

The doctors from group two, who viewed the more dramatic presentation, tended to diagnose anxiety and panic attacks more often than cardiac problems. As a result, they were far less likely to pursue a cardiac workup.

And in the third group, the internists who simply read a transcript of the interview were fairly equally divided between gastrointestinal, cardiac, and psychological diagnoses.[19]

We Often Minimize Our Symptoms.

A particular problem some women have—especially those who suffer from certain chronic diseases—is the tendency to minimize, or even, inadvertently, misrepresent their symptoms. Rachel Kindle, sixty-one, suffers from fibromyalgia, which forced her to leave her position in corporate communications and work from home as a freelance writer and marketing and public relations consultant.

 Approximately ten million people suffer from fibromyalgia. Between 7.5 and 9 million of them are women—that's 75 to 90 percent.[20]

She explains why communication issues are common among fibromyalgia sufferers:

Fibromyalgia is not diagnosable with devices such as X-rays or MRIs. It is symptom-driven, so patients who present poorly, are vague, speak more generally, or are unable to articulate will have a harder time with their physician visits.

My pain is only one part of my illness. A lot of the fibromyalgia sufferers in my support group experience what we call brain or fibro fog, and we mix up our words and numbers. It's easy to feel that the doctor's not listening because what we say is not always clear. It takes a minute to realize that we're the problem.

Desireé Daruma said sometimes the experience of going to the doctor is challenging for lupus patients, too:

If the wait is too long, we often become too tired to describe what's going on. Lupus patients also suffer from brain fog. What happens is that by the time they finally get to see the doctor, they say, "It's OK, the pain comes and goes." They're so tired and fogged up, they just want to go home. So when the doctor says, "Hi, how are you doing?" they say, "Oh, fine."

Most doctors are under tremendous time constraints and have little control over the duration of patient visits. That may be partly why many doctors fail to realize patients are minimizing their discomfort. Nevertheless, it's still surprising that so many doctors don't recognize the problem. For example, in 2012, GfK Roper Public Affairs and Communications surveyed 502 patients diagnosed with lupus. They found that 87 percent of the patients claimed to downplay their symptoms when they talked to their doctor, but 72 percent of the 251 rheumatologists surveyed were unaware their patients did this.[21]

We Even Lie.

The most astonishing thing I came across in my research was how many of us actually lie to our doctors about our symptoms and health habits![22] Of course that's a behavioral issue, not a speech habit or conversational style. But lying occurs much more frequently than I anticipated.

Do any of these statements sound familiar? "Of course, I exercise regularly." "I never forget to take my medications." "I only have one, maybe two drinks on the weekend." "I stopped smoking ages ago." "Sure, I floss twice a day, morning and night."

One study showed that although nearly 80 percent of health care professionals say at least 25 percent of their patients—both men and women—omit facts or downright lie about their personal health, a whopping 52 percent of women routinely "stretch the truth" when they talk to their doctor.[23]

Other times, we don't outright lie, but we withhold information, particularly information that we think could make us look bad.[24] We want to be "good patients" and gain our doctors' approval, and we don't want them to judge, lecture, or criticize us. So we just say to ourselves, "I can't tell my doctor *THAT!*"[25]

Alexandra Nowakowski, a medical sociologist, describes how she wanted to "tough it out" and, as a result, withheld the side effects of a new medication from her doctor:

> I feared that to report side effects would be to report failure—not just of the therapy itself, but also of myself as an individual. . . . I felt a deep sense of failure and shame. . . . Even as the side effects escalated

dramatically, I still wondered if the side effects were all in my head.[26]

Another surprising fact is how strongly we deny that our lies have any implications for our diagnosis or treatment. A national survey reported that more than 25 percent of the women surveyed didn't believe their lies were a big deal and seemed unconcerned that they could result in misdiagnosis and ineffective, or even harmful, treatment.[27]

We even lie about taking our medications. An article in *Consumer Reports on Health* says that many patients (women and men) tell their doctors they're taking their medication as directed, even though they're not.[28] And a study conducted by Dr. Andrea Gurmankin Levy and her colleagues was more specific: they found that approximately 20 percent of the patients in their studies avoided telling their doctors that they failed to take their medication as instructed.[29]

Some Fun Facts

Here are a few other interesting points about patient-doctor communication that are worth thinking about. Most of them are about how *doctors* communicate, and generally they're not gender-specific. But it's easy to see how all of them can affect the quality of the interaction and the patient's understanding of what she is being told.

❖ *Consumer Reports on Health* reveals that, providing they are not interrupted, it can take patients about 90 seconds to describe their symptoms.[30]

Not too bad, you might think. But they also report that patients may only get to speak about 15 to 23 seconds before their doctor interrupts.[31] That may be why 11 percent of patients feel their doctors don't listen.[32]

❖ Dr. Donna Rhoades, from the University of South Carolina, and colleagues write that male doctors seem to interrupt patients more frequently than female doctors.[33]

❖ In their study of 264 physician visits, Dr. Kim Marvel, from the Poudre Valley Health System in Fort Collins, Colorado, and colleagues found most interruptions (76 percent) occur after patients state their first concern. But when physicians redirect the conversation, only 33 percent of patients go on to state any additional concerns. That is particularly unfortunate because once the discussion becomes focused on a specific topic, Marvel reported that only 8 percent of patients went on to complete their full agenda.[34]

❖ In *Doctors Talking with Patients/Patients Talking With Doctors* (2006), Roter and Hall report that only 15 percent of us tell our doctors when we don't understand something. We may feel flattered that our doctors think we're sophisticated enough to grasp what they're saying and hesitate to admit our ignorance by asking for clarification. Other times, we're just too intimidated to ask.[35]

What We Can Do About It

The most important thing you can do is to find a physician you feel comfortable with, one who you feel genuinely likes you and is easy to talk to. But if you already have a doctor who falls short on that front and you're not yet ready to look for someone new, here are some steps you can take to improve your relationship.

❖ Write down a list of questions before your visit, and list the most important questions at the top. The list helps organize your thoughts, it focuses your visit, and it keeps you and your doctor from veering off track. Coming in with a list of questions also helps you assess your doctor's willingness to address them. If there's not enough time to go over all your questions, request a follow-up appointment to continue the conversation.

❖ Don't introduce a new problem at the very end of your visit. Twenty percent of patients make this mistake, and it's unfair to both you and the doctor.[36] A prioritized list that you write before your visit will help you avoid that happening.

❖ Try to repeat back, in your own words, what you hear the doctor saying. If you're like me, I can get so anxious that I find it impossible to hear clearly. Although I'm always a little shy and embarrassed to show that I didn't get it the first time, I often need to have the information repeated at least once, if not more. Repeating back what you hear gives both you

72

In the early 2000s, Dr. Jane Ogden and her colleagues recruited 740 patients, mostly women, and gave them a questionnaire with two fictitious cases: each case described identical stomach and throat problems, but the language used to diagnose the conditions was different.

One case used lay language, such as stomach upset and sore throat; the other used more clinical terminology, such as gastroenteritis and tonsillitis.

It turned out patients preferred the clinical language. They thought it validated them and helped them feel they were *"really* sick" and that their illness was not their fault. They also thought it made the doctor sound more competent.

When doctors used the words "upset stomach" and "sore throat," patients thought it meant the doctors believed they had brought the problem on themselves and should not have sought help. They felt doctors were blaming them and wanted to end the consultation.[37]

and your doctor the opportunity to clarify what's been said.

❖ As the visit progresses, ask any and all questions that occur to you—beyond those on your list.

❖ Try to bring someone with you who can help listen and write down what's said. That way you can concentrate on the conversation without worrying about whether you're getting it all. Patients typically forget between 40 and 80 percent of the information the doctor provides.[38] So the ability to review the doctor's comments at a later date allows you to call back or email to clarify anything you still have questions about.

❖ Always ask for the clinical name of your condition or recommended procedure so you can do your own research. With any medications the doctor prescribes, you'll want to know the scientific name (not just the generic), as well as the appropriate dosage, the length of time to take it, the side effects to watch out for, and the other medications, foods, or drinks with which it may interact.[39] Ask for the medication patient-information handout. And be sure to ask how long it should take for the medicine to work. You don't want to panic after a few days if the drug takes two weeks before it's supposed to kick in.

❖ Last, but not least—and this is something I still have difficulty with—don't be afraid to state how you're truly feeling. It's all too easy to fall into the trap of wanting to be the good patient who doesn't complain. So many people I talked with commented that when their doctor asked them about the severity of their pain, they were dismissive about it and said things like, "It's OK," or, with a shrug, "I'll live," even though they were miserable. When we play that game, we do both ourselves and our doctor a disservice.

Remember, language works when it enables physicians and patients to work together. Then and only then is it doing its job. And it follows that silence—whether on the part of patients or doctors—is rarely golden. In fact, when communication fails, patients often end up making a decision with only half the information they need. To paraphrase Sir Francis Bacon (1561–1626), the English philosopher, author, scientist, and lawyer, silence is often the virtue of fools.

CHAPTER 5

MY BODY, MY SELF

The Role of Emotions in Recovery

S usan Taylor was thirty-three when she begged her doctor for a hysterectomy. For many years she had suffered from endometriosis that caused terrible pain during intercourse and "huge menstrual periods that even Maxi pads didn't help."

Susan's mother had died at fifty from cervical cancer, and Susan was terrified she was following in her mother's footsteps. She requested the hysterectomy to relieve her symptoms and her fears of an early death.

"I talked my doctor into the operation," Susan explained. "I was so knowledgeable about hysterectomies and had thoroughly researched all the technical aspects of the surgery. I probably could have performed it myself," she joked.

The operation did ease Susan's physical symptoms, but it came with an unpleasant and unexpected side effect: her sex drive almost completely disappeared. After two previous marriages that Susan called "a disaster," she had remarried before her hysterectomy. But the surgery caused unexpected difficulties in their relationship. She continued with tears in her eyes:

> I love my husband dearly. I never got anything out of this sexual stuff until I married him. And now . . . I've had no sex drive since my surgery. None. Nothing. It's the emotional part I get starved for, the closeness, that really incredible intimate bond. I'd prepared a list of over thirty-five questions to ask my doctor, but it never occurred to me to think about the surgery's sexual and emotional ramifications. If I had known about those, I might have changed my mind about the operation. I made a huge mistake.

Women who suffer from endometriosis, like Susan, seem to have more post-hysterectomy sexual issues than women whose conditions are more benign. But still, more than 20 percent of women who have the surgery report some measure of deteriorated sexual function.[1]

Like Beth Tiner, Jill Essex, a high school teacher in Madison, Wisconsin, found herself totally surprised by how seriously depressed she became after her surgery. She, too, felt something was wrong with her:

> I wasn't prepared for how much the hormones would affect my emotions and screw up my head. I thought there was something wrong with me.

Everyone has a hysterectomy and gets over it. What's the matter with me?

As Jill said, because of the nature of her surgery, her depression was more than likely hormonal. Nevertheless, her reaction surprised her. And many patients experience depression after any kind of operation for reasons no one completely understands. There are a variety of possibilities, including the anesthesia or just the general trauma of surgery. But feelings of vulnerability, anxiety, and depression are so common after illness and surgery that the website Medical News Today offers a list of those surgeries that carry a high postoperative depression rate:[2]

- ❖ Heart surgery
- ❖ Gastric bypass surgery
- ❖ Brain surgery
- ❖ Hip replacement
- ❖ Hysterectomy
- ❖ Cancer resection
- ❖ Mastectomy
- ❖ Plastic surgery

Why Are Emotions So Important to Recovery?

Susan and Jill weren't the only women I spoke with who didn't consider the possibility that their illness could have serious emotional repercussions. In fact, most of the women I interviewed said it never occurred to them. I found that odd because, as I discussed in the previous chapter, we seem to have no problem letting our emotions play a central role when describing our *symptoms* to a doctor. In fact, our tendency to describe in detail how we *feel* about what's going on is often at odds with the doctor's more clinical approach, and sometimes that clash of communication can make it difficult to get the right diagnosis.

But I found that when it comes to selecting a treatment or thinking about our recovery, our emotions fall by the wayside. We treat our minds and bodies as two separate entities and don't always think about their effect on each other. It's not that we're unaware that our minds and bodies are connected. Perhaps it comes back to that other problem we often have, of putting ourselves second. If we need to take care of our families and keep up with our work responsibilities, we can't really afford to worry about anything but getting the quickest relief possible. It's bad enough to be out of commission because of physical pain or discomfort; who wants to consider the possibility that they might feel better physically but still be held back by annoying and amorphous emotional problems?

But minimizing emotions can have serious repercussions for our recovery, propelling us into a negative cycle that works something like this: We're sick and don't feel well, which, of course, stresses us out. But we try to keep going and fulfill our various responsibilities. Then, like Jill Essex, because we weren't expecting to feel so stressed, we may blame ourselves for whining or complaining.

Now we're ashamed of how poorly we think we're dealing with our situation, and our shame and guilt stresses us out even more. Rather than focus our energy just on getting

The mind and the body were once considered so connected that Asclepius, the god of medicine, carried a staff symbolizing them intertwined. It was a wooden staff with a serpent curled around it, an ancient symbol of body and soul. Today it is the universally recognized symbol of medicine.[3]

better, we also worry about feeling bad about ourselves for having such an emotionally hard time. And because we're so sure that we're the problem, we may be too embarrassed to call the doctor and get some relief. Remember Alexandra Nowakowski, the medical sociologist I described in the previous chapter, who felt that reporting side effects to her doctor meant she was admitting a personal failure?

Our Minds and Bodies Work Together

When we treat our minds and bodies as separate entities, we're ignoring decades of research and observation that show that we shouldn't. Here are two fun experiments that illustrate just how strong the body-mind link is. While they're not specifically about that connection in relation to illness, their implications carry over.

Researchers from the Massachusetts Institute of Technology, Harvard, and Yale asked fifty-four people to evaluate job candidates by reviewing their resumes on either light or heavy clipboards. The participants using the heavier clipboards rated their candidates as "heavyweights," better overall, and more seriously interested in the position than participants using the lighter clipboards.[4]

And here's my favorite: In 2008, Yale researchers divided college students into two groups, took them into different rooms, and casually offered each group some coffee. The coffee for the first group was hot; for the second, it was iced. As they drank their coffee, the students were given the same packet of information about a fictitious person and asked to evaluate the "person's" personality. Those students holding the warm coffee were far likelier to judge the fictitious person as warm and likable than the group holding the iced coffee.[5]

And what we think affects our bodies just as much as the other way around. One more fun experiment for you: Researchers at the University of Toronto asked a group of sixty-five students to remember a time when they had felt either socially accepted or rejected. Those students who remembered feeling rejected judged the temperature of the room where the study was taking place to be approximately 5 degrees cooler than those who were basking in the warm, fuzzy thoughts of social acceptance.[6]

This next study not only clearly establishes the mind-body link; it also happens to be a couch potato's dream: In the early 2000s, researchers from the Cleveland Clinic wanted to find out whether people could become stronger just by mentally visualizing an exercise—that is, *without* actually performing it. They recruited four groups of volunteers, mostly men. Two of the groups were randomly assigned mental training only—no physical exercise at all.

The participants in the first group were told to try to strengthen their little finger; those in the second group were told to work on their biceps. During each training session, participants in both groups were instructed to *imagine* their finger or forearm pushing maximally against the force transducer that was to measure their strength. (A transducer is a device that converts one physical quantity into another.) The participants were instructed to adopt an approach in which they urged their muscles to contract as much as possible. The researchers called the process "visualization-guided brain activation."

Group three engaged in actual physical training of their biceps and their little fingers.

Group four, the control group, was told to do nothing different. Training lasted twelve weeks.

The results are astonishing. As expected, the physical training group increased their finger strength substantially, by 56 percent. But surprisingly, the finger strength of the mental training group increased by 35 percent. Four weeks after the training ended, it jumped to 40 percent.

The bicep group also saw an increase in strength, though it was significantly less than what the finger group experienced: 13.5 percent. The researchers attributed this difference to the fact that our little fingers are weaker than our biceps to begin with, so they have more room for improvement.

Group four, the control group, experienced no changes.

All the participants underwent an EEG to record the electrical activity of their brains, and the results showed that the visualization alone changed their brain activity. The researchers concluded that visualization enhanced the central command to the muscles and trained and enabled the brain to generate stronger signals.[7]

The Stress/Sickness Connection

It's just a small leap from understanding how powerfully our minds can influence our bodies to understanding why unexpected stressful emotions can make us sick or complicate our recovery. How many times have you said to yourself, or heard someone say, "I always get a cold during the holidays" or "I wish I could take exams without getting headaches"? Although the research is mixed, women are thought to be more vulnerable to these effects than men are.[8]

 Feeling ill can be a strong cry for help and is a culturally accepted way of expressing frustration and grief. Dr. Laurence J. Kirmayer in the Division of Social and Transcultural Psychiatry at McGill University believes that "somatic symptoms are the most common clinical expression of emotional distress worldwide."[9]

Physicians were aware of how strongly our minds influence how we feel physically as far back as ancient Greece. A medical practitioner named Erasistratus (310–250 BCE) was asked to consult in a particularly difficult case about a seriously ill young man, Antiochus. The family had tried many different doctors, but no one could figure out what was going on. Erasistratus was the family's last resort.

He observed his patient carefully and analyzed his physiological reactions to the various people who visited. He noticed that each time Antiochus's stepmother showed up, Antiochus stammered and blushed, became pale, and had palpitations. He "diagnosed" that Antiochus was in love with his stepmother, and his efforts to hide it were making him sick. Erasistratus believed that we can consciously choose to conceal our thoughts but that we can't control how they affect our bodies. In a sense, he invented love sickness. (Unfortunately, the story doesn't report how he treated it.)[10]

A corollary to "love sickness" is what we might call "stress sickness," a more contemporary phenomenon. Dr. Jeff Huffman, director of the Cardiac Psychiatry Research Program at Massachusetts General Hospital, says that our state of mind can affect our recovery from a physical setback. When we're under stress, our fight-or-flight response goes into overdrive, which can raise blood pressure and trigger inflammation, which can make recovery longer and more difficult. Dr. Huffman adds, "And mild depression related to our setback can weaken the motivation and attention we need to take better care of ourselves."[11]

In 2011, for example, Ohio State University researchers gave a small group of women a "punch biopsy," a low-risk dermatology technique, in their forearm that created a small wound. The wounds of women who were stressed from taking care of family members with dementia took approximately nine days (or 24 percent) longer to heal than the wounds of women who were non-caregivers.[12]

In *The Balance Within* (2001), Dr. Esther Sternberg, at the Center for Integrative Medicine at the University of Arizona, explains some of the physiology behind this phenomenon:

The same parts of the brain that control the stress response, for example, play an important role in susceptibility and resistance to inflammatory diseases such as arthritis. And since it is these parts of the brain that also play a role in depression, we can begin to understand why it is that many patients with inflammatory disease may also experience depression.[13]

Indeed, research from the American Heart Association found that 20 percent of cardiovascular disease patients suffer from depression, which can affect how well they deal with their condition. The researchers noted that heart attack patients diagnosed with depression were 54 percent more likely to be hospitalized compared to those who weren't depressed.[14] (Heart surgery was on the list of those surgeries that carry a high postoperative depression rate.)

Fun fact: Gray whales are one of the longest-lived mammals, and their secret seems to be their resilience to stress.

Dimitri Toren and his colleagues from the Romanian Academy in Bucharest investigate aging, and in one of their experiments, they took biopsies of liver and kidney tissue from two gray whales. They found that, on a molecular level, the whales were able to maintain and repair the DNA involved in the immune system and were able to flush out damaged proteins.

Lorna Harris at the University of Exeter in the UK says that our molecular stress response tends to decline with age. If we can maintain our stress response, chances are we'll age better.[15]

Interestingly, coping with anxiety or depression *before* we have a procedure or surgery also affects how well or easily we recover from it. According to a study in the *British Journal of Surgery*, researchers reviewed the health information of 177,000 people who had undergone hip and knee replacements, hernia repairs, and varicose vein operations. They found that the likelihood of experiencing complications was 17 percent greater among those diagnosed with moderate anxiety or depression *prior to* the surgery. These patients also had a 20 percent greater chance of readmission to the hospital because of their wounds.[16]

The Gut-Brain Axis

One of the most exciting areas of research suggests yet another pathway in the body/mind connection. We're coming to understand more and more about how the bacteria in our guts can influence our emotions. An unbalanced gut can make us feel anxious; a well-balanced one can improve our moods. In *New Scientist*, Scott Anderson, a science journalist and one of the authors of *The Psychobiotic Revolution* (2017), writes,

> Remember the last time you had a stomach bug and just wanted to crawl into bed and pull up the covers? This is called "sickness-behavior" and it's a kind of short-term depression. The bacteria infecting you aren't just making you feel nauseous; they are controlling your mood.[17]

According to dietician Dr. Megan Rossi, a research fellow at King's College London, people who have at least thirty plant-based elements in their weekly diet have a more diverse range of bacteria in their gut. As a result, they have better weight management, better heart health, and better mental health.[19]

The gut microbiota—the trillions of microorganisms in our guts—and the connection between microbes and mood is called the "gut-brain axis," and it has been implicated in schizophrenia, autism, anxiety and, major depressive disorders.[18]

Placebos: When Our Feelings *Help* Us Heal

Fortunately, there's another side to the mind-body coin that can work to our advantage. Our minds and bodies are so connected that between 30 and 40 percent of patients get better when they take a placebo. The word *placebo* comes from Latin and means "I will please." It's a "drug" that contains no actual medicine, and no one knows exactly how or why it works.[20] But placebos show the positive effects that can come from how people think about the treatment they're having.[21]

Placebos have been around a long time. Galen (139–201 CE), a Greek physician in the Roman Empire, believed that the patient's degree of trust in their doctor was more important for their healing than the particular treatment he recommended.

Hundreds of years later, even Thomas Jefferson reflected on the power of placebos: "One of the most successful physicians I know has assured me that he used more bread pills, drops of colored water, and powders of hickory ashes, than of all other medicines put together."[22]

The placebo effect is even apparent in pop culture—think of *The Wizard of Oz*. While the wizard faked his skills, his mind tricks helped characters who were ailing in one way or another to feel better. That's what placebos are all about.[23]

Some people still dismiss placebos as pure silliness, more myth than medicine. In *Hippocrates' Shadow* (2008), Dr. David Newman, from Columbia University and St. Luke's Roosevelt Hospital Center, even says that some people think we fall for the placebo effect just because we're gullible.

But that's not true. There's an actual physiological mechanism at play. It turns out that when we *expect* something to happen, nerves get stimulated, biochemical changes occur, internal substances are released, and pain is relieved.[24] Here are some interesting findings from some of the placebo research:

- ❖ Two placebos work better than one.[25]
- ❖ Capsules are more effective than pills, and large capsules work better than smaller ones.[26]
- ❖ Pink or red placebo pills seem to have stimulant effects; blue placebo pills tend to act as sedatives. Green pills seem to be the most effective for anxiety.[27]
- ❖ Placebo injections are more effective than placebo capsules and pills, and they seem to be more effective in women than they are in men.[28]
- ❖ Old placebo drugs seem to become less effective after new ones come along. It isn't necessarily that

the new placebo drugs are better than the old ones; some research suggests that it's just because people *perceive* them to be.[29]

❖ Sugar pills and saline injections have been shown to relieve pain, anxiety, and depression. They can also reduce tremors in Parkinson's, lower blood pressure, and open up airways in patients with asthma.[30]

❖ When placebo back pain medication is given by a human being, patients need much less of it than when it is dispensed automatically by an infusion machine, unless it's a machine that emits sounds and has blinking lights. When that's the case, the machines are actually more effective than a person.[31]

Nocebos: When Our Feelings *Hinder* How We Heal

Placebos have an evil twin, nocebos, whose name comes from the Latin and means "I will harm." The nocebo effect simply means that expecting the worst means you're likely to *experience* the worst. And it's observed more in women than in men.[32] Just anticipating pain, for example, can cause some women to perceive non-painful stimulation as painful and low-painful stimulation as highly painful.[33] Or if your friend became nauseated and depressed from taking a certain drug, because of your friend's experience, you may well be too preconditioned against taking it to gain any of its benefits. When people talk about being "scared to death" and "worried sick," they're actually describing the nocebo effect.

The nocebo effect has been known to induce symptoms as varied as facial swelling, rashes, dizziness, dry mouth, nausea, and diarrhea.[34] In some cases, it can even be fatal. Brian Reid, who writes about health for the *Washington Post*, reports that surgeons dislike operating on patients who want to die because their chances of dying are much higher.[35]

What We Can Do About It

It can be difficult to learn how to deal with pain and discomfort, especially if we're also dealing with the stress of being unable to care for ourselves or our families.[36] Whatever the reasons, there are some things you can do:

❖ Particularly if you're having surgery, be sure you understand the entire picture, such as the sexual or psychological effects of the procedure. Remember Susan Taylor, and don't be taken by surprise. Know what to expect.

❖ Don't hesitate to call your doctors if things come up that you *didn't* talk about. Ask if these feelings are typical and what you should do about them.

❖ Reach out to friends and family so that you feel supported.

❖ If you have access to a computer, go on the Internet and see what other women have to say about your disease or procedure. More than likely, you'll find a list of support groups of women you can join with a similar disease or who had a similar surgery. It can be helpful to find out how others feel and what, if anything, they did to help themselves feel better. Maybe they did nothing, and as time passed, their feelings subsided. That can be very useful for you to know.

❖ Be patient. Give yourself some time to recover. Feeling frustrated isn't helpful.

So many of us view sickness as more a matter of the cell than the soul.[37] But our minds and bodies aren't structured as separate apartments within a single building. We're more like a small community in which each part is connected and inter-dependent. As with any community, it thrives only when we recognize that *all* of its components work best when working together.

CHAPTER 6

PILLS FOR EVERY ILL

Captives of the Pharmaceutical Industry

Doctors pour medicines about which they know little, for diseases about which they know less, into human beings about whom they know nothing.

—Voltaire

Every day, Desireé Daruma takes hydroxychloroquine and CellCept to treat her lupus; nifedipine, a calcium channel blocker for Raynaud's disease; an aspirin for her heart; fish oil; and a variety of multivitamins for her general health. Beth Tiner takes Synthroid, a synthetic thyroid hormone; Bi-Est, a bioidentical hormone for menopause symptoms; progesterone; testosterone hormones; and tramadol, an opioid, once every other week for pain. Margaret Adams takes Celebrex (an anti-inflammatory) twice a day, tramadol three to four times a day, and a host of other drugs as needed to relieve her fatigue and joint pain from Sjögren's syndrome.

It may sound like a lot, but Desireé, Beth, and Margaret are not unusual in the number of prescription drugs they take. In 2017, *Consumer Reports* revealed that more than half of all Americans take an average of four prescription drugs every day, a number that's risen significantly over the last two decades. Even though our population has increased by only 21 percent, Americans today fill 85 percent *more* prescriptions than ever before, and on average, each of us spends a minimum of four thousand dollars on prescription drugs every year.[1]

In the United States and Canada, just under sixteen million people older than sixty-five take ten or more pills per day.

Just under thirty-nine million people take five or more pills a day.

Just under eighteen million older adults filled prescriptions that the American Geriatrics Society recommends they avoid because they can lead to more harm than good.[2]

Why Are Women Prescribed More Pills Than Men?

At the 2012 Women's Health Conference in Washington, DC, researchers presented a study that examined the prescription and insurance records for approximately sixteen thousand women and fourteen thousand men for the year 2010. They found that women were prescribed an average of five medications during the study period compared to an average of 3.7 for the men. Even *without* contraception, just under 70 percent of the women received prescriptions for at least one medication for a chronic or acute condition compared to less than 60 percent of the men.[3]

There are many reasons for this gender discrepancy. Although we may put ourselves in second place, we visit the doctor more frequently than men, even apart from pregnancy. We're also conditioned early on to believe that preventive care is important, and many of us stay on top of our annual checkups, mammograms, pap smears, etc.[4] (Of course, drug companies are well aware of all of this imbalance and target their ads accordingly.) Obviously, keeping on top of our health care is good to do, but doctor appointments also tend to lead to more prescriptions.

We also suffer disproportionately from certain diseases. As I mentioned earlier, we're more likely than men to have chronic diseases and pain, and we're twice as likely to suffer from anxiety and depression, conditions that are often treated, at least in part, with drugs.

There's no question that many of these drugs are beneficial and can offer tremendous relief from a variety of symptoms. The problem arises when drugs become our default strategy. When that happens, we may end up exposing ourselves to unnecessary side effects, and women are generally more susceptible to side effects than men are. Overdosing is another major issue that affects us more than men.

Normal Conditions Are
Treated as Medical Issues

Part of the problem is that our culture (and again, the drug companies) treats a lot of normal health conditions as medical issues. In 2001, Drs. Steve Woloshin and Lisa Schwartz, codirectors of Medicine and the Media Programs at the Dartmouth Institute for Health Policy and Clinical Practice, and their colleagues analyzed seventy drug company ads in ten popular US men's and women's magazines in 1998 and 1999. They found that approximately 39 percent of the ads encouraged people to consider medical causes for their common experiences and frequently urged them to consult a physician.

The ads posed questions like, "Is it just forgetfulness, or is it Alzheimer's?" "If your heartburn is persistent and occurs on two or more days a week, you probably don't have ordinary heartburn. You may have a potentially serious condition called acid reflux disease." Even sneezing was described as something that might be worthy of a doctor visit.[5]

A year later, *The British Medical Journal* asked their readers to identify issues that people have labeled disease. Here's some of what they said:

❖ Aging
❖ Work
❖ Boredom
❖ Bags under eyes
❖ Baldness
❖ Freckles

❖ Big ears

❖ Grey or white hair

❖ Ugliness

❖ Ignorance

❖ [And my favorite:] Allergy to the twenty-first century[6]

Some of these may seem like jokes, but Woloshin and Schwartz warn of the problem that can result from defining disease so broadly: "The danger is that by turning ordinary experiences into diagnoses—by designating a runny nose as allergic rhinitis—the boundaries of medicine might become unreasonably broad."[7]

Today, if little Miss Muffet were happily eating a snack on her tuffet until a spider scared her away, she may well be diagnosed with arachnophobia, prescribed anti-anxiety medication, or advised to undergo some intensive exposure therapy.

Insomnia is a good example of what can happen when a normal condition is treated like a medical one. According to the Society for Women's Health Research, women are generally 40 percent more likely to experience insomnia than men are. As many as one in four women have some trouble falling asleep, staying asleep, or both. The hormonal changes common in pregnancy and during menstrual cycles and menopause can all cause sleep problems, as can some of the chronic diseases we suffer such as depression, anxiety, and fibromyalgia.

In her 2016 *New Yorker* article "In Search of Forty Winks: Gizmos for a Good Night's Sleep," Patricia Marx describes some of the more outlandish remedies that have been tried throughout the ages to overcome sleep problems. The Romans, for example, smeared mouse fat on the souls of their feet to help them sleep. Charles Dickens could only sleep if he positioned himself in the precise center of a bed that faced exactly north. And in 1879, a Canadian medical journal recommended hemlock as a sleep aid. That sleep might have been longer than one would hope, and, as Marx suggested, "Presumably no repeating was required."[8]

Today, we're still looking for ways to cure insomnia, and drugs are one of the more common remedies in the US, especially for women. Women use more sleep drugs than men: CVS Pharmacy, for example, reports that over 70 percent of their customers for Ambien, a common sleep medication, are women; just over 28 percent are men.

But is insomnia really a medical issue? And are drugs the best way to relieve it? In some cases, yes. Trouble sleeping can be a symptom of a more serious underlying condition, and it's definitely worth checking with a doctor if it becomes chronic. Even if it's not indicative of something worse, the frustration of not being able to get to sleep or stay asleep, and the reverberations that sleeplessness can have in our daily lives, can be upsetting enough to make us want to reach for a pill.[9]

However, no sleep medication is safe enough to take indefinitely on a daily basis. And for many of them, the dose needs to be continually increased for the medication to keep working. So it's always wise to explore other proven alternatives—cognitive behavioral therapy, relaxation tapes, biofeedback, deep breathing, acupuncture—before getting into the habit of taking a drug.

We're Treated for Issues Before
We "Officially" Have Them

In addition to medicating what most of us used to consider normal conditions, the notion of what's treatable now seems to include things for which we only *might* be at risk. The boundaries between "the sick," the "not yet sick," and the "worried well" have become looser and looser. Of course no one would argue with the adage that an ounce of prevention is worth a pound of cure. But 45 percent of American adults (men and women) have been diagnosed with "pre-diseases," diseases they don't yet have.[10] That can happen when screening results aren't quite normal but are still below the threshold for disease. Many people who are diagnosed with pre-diseases think of themselves as sick instead of simply in a phase of watchful waiting for what *could* happen someday. In one study, 100 percent of the participants diagnosed with borderline high blood pressure or prediabetes described themselves as actually having the disease[11]—certainly a good situation for pharmaceutical companies, but not necessarily so for patients.

Consumer Reports published an article in the *Washington Post* that acknowledges while it can be dangerous to ignore warning signs, many treatments come with risks that may outweigh their benefits. For example, prediabetes affects eighty-four million Americans, about one-third of the country. But only 2 percent of those people go on to develop full-blown diabetes each year. It turns out that 17 to 59 percent of people diagnosed as prediabetic reverted to normal blood sugar levels without medication. It's likely that people who are labeled prediabetic may be more motivated to implement the lifestyle changes necessary to improve their blood sugar levels. However, the point is that some of these people may consider themselves ill and go on to take medications that could be unnecessary. In fact, *Consumer Reports* states that scientists found that aggressive treatment for diabetes resulted in a higher death rate than standard care.

Prehypertension affects one in three Americans. But new treatment guidelines recommend medication only if, because of other factors, a person is at high risk for a heart attack or stroke. In fact, the American College of Physicians recommends blood pressure medication only for people over sixty if their systolic pressure (the upper number) is 150 mm Hg or higher.

And one more: Osteopenia, when bone density is below normal but above the threshold for osteoporosis, affects more than forty-three million adults, mostly women. But a 2012 analysis of 4,957 older women found that after fifteen years, only 5 percent went on to develop full-blown osteoporosis. *Consumer Reports* quotes Teppo Järvinen, a professor of orthopedics at the University of Helsinki, who says that bone density itself is actually a relatively weak risk factor for fractures.[12]

That's why Dr. Atul Gawande, a surgeon, public health researcher, and professor in both the Department of Health Policy and Management at the Harvard School of Public Health and the Department of Surgery at the Harvard Medical

School, worries about the consequences of such overly broad definitions of illness. In "Overkill," an article he wrote for *The New Yorker*, he says research indicates that virtually every family in the country has been subject to overtesting and overtreatment in one form or another. While he doesn't say whether women are more at risk for this than men, he is convinced that the problem is huge:

> Millions of people are receiving drugs that aren't helping them, operations that aren't going to make them better, and scans and tests that do nothing beneficial for them and often cause harm.[13]

Dr. Gawande reports that our country of three hundred million people undergoes fifteen million nuclear medicine scans, one hundred million CT and MRI scans, and almost ten billion laboratory tests each year. Often, he says, these are fishing expeditions, and since no one is perfectly normal, you tend to find a lot of fish.[14]

Of course, the pharmaceutical industry bears a great deal of responsibility for this problem. The United States and New Zealand are the only two countries in the world that allow pharmaceutical companies to advertise directly to consumers. In 2020, Statista.com reported that in the first nine months of 2019, pharmaceutical companies spent upward of $4.54 *billion* dollars on consumer advertising alone. That's a jump of approximately 50 percent since 2012.[15] We should all be concerned by that statistic, but women especially so, since we're the primary targets of these ads. And the companies are doing all they can to hone their message to us.

Pharmaceutical Ads Target Women

One study reviewed ninety-seven direct-to-consumer ads for prescription drugs broadcast in the United States from January 2015 to July 2016 and found that the majority have female protagonists.[16] The ads are carefully designed to make us anxious and insecure—about our bodies, our behavior, our children's behavior, etc.—and then to persuade us that help is possible if we just purchase whatever drug the company is promoting.[17]

They also target our caretaking role because research shows that women respond well to claims that a particular medication will help us help others.[18] Many ads specifically exploit our desire and ability to be good mothers. In the September 2018 issue of *Redbook*, an ad for Enbrel, a drug for rheumatoid arthritis, shows a mother and child with the caption, "Since Enbrel, my mom's back to being mom." With guilt trips like this, it's no wonder women take the bait.

And these ads have been wildly successful. In 2003, Dr. Barbara Mintzes, a research scientist specializing in pharmaceutical policy, and her colleagues recruited 78 primary care physicians from Sacramento, California, and Vancouver, Canada, and 1,431 adult patients from both cities. The majority of the physicians were male, and the patients were divided more or less equally between men and women. Not surprisingly, Dr. Mintzes found that the more ads patients were exposed to, the more drugs they requested from their doctors. In fact, according to the Congressional Budget Office

According to Kantar Media:

Two-thirds of adults take some kind of action after seeing a drug ad.

Forty percent make an appointment with their doctor.

Seventy-six percent of people feel drug companies adequately explain side effects and risks.

Forty-three percent of Americans think only completely safe drugs are allowed to be advertised.[20]

and Kantar Media, a research and data company, in 2011, drugs that had been advertised to consumers had nine times more prescriptions written than those that weren't.[19]

What we may not realize when we request drugs we've seen advertised is that the ads are not necessarily trustworthy. Dr. Adrienne E. Faerber, a researcher at the Dartmouth Institute for Health Policy and Clinical Practice, and Dr. David Kreling from the Sonderegger Research Center at the University of Wisconsin analyzed television drug advertising from 2008 to 2010. They found that overall, only 33 percent of the advertised claims were true, 57 percent were potentially misleading, and 10 percent were completely false. They report that in some cases, information was exaggerated, and in others, important facts were simply omitted.[21] The ads also tended to minimize negative information. Side effects, for example, were generally listed either very rapidly or in very small type and often conflicted with the visual on the screen.

A 2017 television commercial for Lyrica, a drug intended to relieve fibromyalgia symptoms, is a good example of this.

In it, a depressed-looking woman is standing and watching two children play. As you watch, your assumption will be that the woman is their mother and that she is in too much pain to play with them. Then, a glorious garden fills the television screen, and the "patient" is suddenly watering and arranging roses with her "daughter." At the same time, a voice-over says that suicidal thoughts and tendencies are a possible side effect.[22] The visual makes it hard to take the suicide warnings seriously.

Healthnewsreview.org describes the "picture-superiority effect": As drug companies well know, the picture-superiority effect means that advertising that shows imagery is much more likely to be remembered by consumers than advertising that uses words alone. And that's why drug advertisers use imagery so heavily.

Another Lyrica ad shows a different depressed woman (even her dog looks depressed) who was unable to participate in daily life until she took the drug. After she did, the visuals in the ad imply that she is now a happy, satisfied, and fully functioning adult.[23] While the ad lists the serious side effects that Lyrica can cause, they stand in stark contrast to the visuals.

In a 2017 article in the *New York Times*, Joanne Kaufman quotes Maryann Kuzel, executive vice president of Global Health Strategy, Data, and Analytics at Publicis Health, a healthcare communications agency, who says that these exhaustive lists of possible side effects can also become white noise; people stop hearing them.[24] Equally troubling, though, is that the lists can also have the opposite effect. According to the same *New York Times* article, Jeff Rothstein, the chief executive officer of CultHealth, an ad agency specializing in healthcare, says that all that information sometimes makes people trust the ads even more. Howard Courtemanche, president of the health and wellness practice at Young & Rubicam, agrees, saying that people start thinking, "I'm in a serious situation here and I need a very strong drug. Of course there are side effects."[25]

One way or the other, the pharmaceutical companies seem to be winning the game, and as women, we're in danger of losing big.

Consumers (women *and* men) aren't solely responsible for the huge success of direct-to-consumer ads. Dr. Mintzes and her colleagues found that when we request specific medications, some of our doctors may be a bit too willing to accommodate us. Even though many doctors believe the ads encourage patients to seek unnecessary treatment, patients who requested a particular prescription drug were much more likely to receive it than those who made no request at all.[26]

In a 2014 study, Dr. John B. McKinlay, from the New England Research Institutes, and his colleagues recruited 192 primary care physicians from six states. They made videos using professional actors to portray patients with two common, painful conditions: sciatica, where pain radiates along the path of the sciatic nerve that branches from your lower back through your hips and buttocks and down each leg, and chronic knee osteoarthritis.

Half the "patients" with sciatica symptoms requested oxycodone, a strong opioid pain medication; the other half requested "something to help with pain." Similarly, half of the knee osteoarthritis "patients" requested Celebrex, a non-steroidal anti-inflammatory drug (NSAID), while the other half requested "something to help with pain." The medications the "patients" requested were carefully chosen to be plausible choices.

The results are shocking. It turned out that close to 20 percent of the sciatica patients received the prescription for the oxycodone that they had requested, compared to only 1 percent of those who made no specific request. Even if the patients who asked for oxycodone didn't receive it, they were more likely to be prescribed a stronger narcotic than those who simply asked for a pain reliever.

Also, while only 24 percent of the osteoarthritis patients who made no specific request received a prescription for Celebrex, 53 percent of the patients who requested Celebrex received it. While Celebrex is recommended for arthritis treatment, it's more expensive than other options and is no more helpful.

The researchers speculated that one reason for this discrepancy is that physicians genuinely want to respect patients' autonomy and take their concerns seriously.[27] Indeed, ProCon, a non-profit organization that researches controversial issues, reports that 50 percent of patients who were denied the drug they requested were disappointed with their doctors. Twenty-five percent said they would try to obtain the drug elsewhere, and 15 percent said they would change doctors altogether.[28]

I think, too, that the advent of Yelp and other customer-satisfaction surveys has meant that patients now have a public forum in which to express their opinions, which may, in turn, be subtly (or not so subtly) pressuring some doctors to be more accommodating. Furthermore, *Consumer Reports* suggests that for increasingly harried healthcare professionals, dashing off a prescription can be the easiest and quickest way to address patients' concerns.

Women Often Don't Comply with Their Doctor's Instructions

Women often don't follow through with their physician's instructions. And I think that's another factor that may influence doctors to prescribe the medications their patients request: research shows that 20 to 30 percent of medication prescriptions are never filled, and approximately 50 percent of medications for chronic disease are not taken as prescribed. Jane Brody, Personal Health columnist for the *New York Times*, calls non-adherence to prescribed medications an out-of-control epidemic in the United States. In fact, an article in the 2016 *Journal of the American Osteopathic Association* was titled "Medical Noncompliance: The Most Ignored National Epidemic."[29] Brody writes that lack of adherence is estimated to cause approximately 125,000 deaths each year.[30] With that dire statistic in mind, doctors may feel that patients might be more likely to comply if they prescribe the medication their patients request.

However, none of this changes the fact that pharmaceutical ads are having a profound effect on doctors' prescribing practices, and since women are the primary audience for these ads, we're the ones most likely to request and be offered these drugs.

"Drugs don't work in patients who don't take them."

—attributed to C. Everett Koop, MD, former US surgeon general

Nevertheless, there are some good reasons women may hesitate to take the drugs their doctors prescribe. One reason is that we suffer more side effects from medications than men. That's because for years, women were simply excluded from most clinical studies of medications, and there's just not as much known about how our bodies react to drugs. Yet it seems obvious that women and men would have different responses. Prescription guidelines, for example, are generally gender blind even though many side effects are dose-related.[31] So even though the average woman is smaller than the average man, at standard drug doses, we receive a higher amount per body weight than men. We also metabolize medications differently because we have a higher percentage of body fat and more hormonal fluctuations. And there are gender differences in liver metabolism and kidney function as well.[32]

In some instances, researchers said they omitted women from clinical trials because they were trying to protect women who might become pregnant during the trials from potentially

Women make up half the population, but in neuroscience studies, males outnumber females approximately six to one.[33]

negative consequences.[34] Another rationale, however, was that all those pesky female hormones would muddy the study results, and focusing on men alone would make for a "cleaner" analysis. According to Dr. Daniela Pollak, a neurobiologist in Vienna, "The problem is that this assumption sets up men as the norm." So history repeats itself, and males have become the current standard or the reference population.[35]

 Just under 132 million Americans belong to a racial or ethnic minority. Even though the symptoms of many diseases vary across ethnicities, the patients who participate in clinical trials are still primarily white.[36]

But even when women were included in clinical trials, as long ago as 1992, the federal General Accounting Office reported that pharmaceutical manufacturers were not analyzing their data for gender differences. So if women experienced more or different adverse reactions than men, that fact went unreported.

The end result is that women's bodies are less well understood than men's, which is why, as early as 1985, the US Public Health Service Task Force on Women's Health Issues issued the following warning:

The historical lack of research focus on women's health concerns has compromised the quality of health information available to women as well as the health care they receive.[37]

Take Ambien, for example, available in regular and controlled doses. It provides a textbook case of the different effects the same dose of a drug can have on women and men. Ambien was tested mostly on men, and for years the recommended dosage was 10 mg for both genders. But because women's bodies process Ambien more slowly than men's, its effects last longer in us. Researchers found that after eight hours, a 10 mg dose of regular Ambien impaired the abilities of 15 percent of women the next morning, compared with only 3 percent of men.[38] Besides possibly causing headaches, dizziness, and drowsiness that lasted through the day, it also nearly doubled people's risk for car accidents, a particular danger that was seen in both women *and* men.[39] In 2013, the Food and Drug Administration finally recommended that women cut their dosage of Ambien in half for both the regular and controlled-release versions.

Overdosing is another major issue for women. The National Institute on Drug Abuse reports that women are at greater risk than men for mental health and sleep issues such as depression, anxiety, and insomnia. And the drugs prescribed for these conditions, antidepressants and benzodiazepines (anti-anxiety or sleep drugs), can be habit forming when taken regularly or in large quantities.

Another problem is that more women than men receive opioid prescriptions. One reason is we're often prescribed opioids for chronic conditions such as headaches and other pain. Yet research shows that opioids are not highly effective for treating chronic pain; in fact, over time, they can actually cause increased sensitivity to it.[40]

Obviously, overdoses can be fatal. The CDC reports that for men and women, prescription opioids were involved in

35 percent of all opioid overdose deaths. In fact, while more men than women die from prescription opioids, the rate of increase in deaths is higher in women than in men. Between 1999 and 2016, opioid deaths rose by 583 percent in women, compared to 404 percent in men. Particularly alarming is that women who overdose are less likely than men to get life-saving treatment on the way to an emergency department. A study of 124 opioid overdoses in Rhode Island found that paramedics were three times more likely to give men medication to reverse opioid effects than they were women.[41] That could be one reason why former CDC Director, Dr. Thomas Frieden, commented that more women are dying from adverse drug reactions than ever.[42]

What We Can Do About It

First and foremost, we need to become even more discerning consumers. That means taking drug advertisements you read or see in magazines, in television ads, and on the Internet with a BIG grain of salt. Researching a medication yourself is helpful, of course, but more importantly, that research should become the starting point for a discussion with your doctor, not something you present to her with your mind made up.

But even doctors don't necessarily have, or may not offer, all the information you need. *UCLA Magazine* reported in 2007 that, generally speaking, doctors instructed only 55 percent of patients about appropriate dosages, told patients how long to use medications only 34 percent of the time, and noted the frequency or timing of doses only 58 percent of the time.[43] They addressed side effects with their patients for only 35 percent of the medications they prescribed.[44] (The instructions were clearer for psychiatric and pain medications, perhaps because they have the potential for serious adverse effects.)

In addition to asking about all those things, *Consumer Reports* has some specific suggestions for managing medications that I found helpful:

❖ Don't rush into taking drugs too quickly. It's always wise to check into any lifestyle changes you could make first.[45]

❖ If you're taking medication prescribed from more than one doctor, designate one doctor to oversee all of your meds.

❖ Be sure to tell your doctor about any over-the-counter drugs or dietary supplements, including liquids, pills, drops, and ointments, that you take regularly.

❖ If you are taking more than one drug to treat the same health problem, you might be taking a drug you don't need. Ask your doctor to regularly review your drug regimen with you.

❖ If you need one drug to control the side effects of another (for example, if you take a laxative to ease constipation caused by another drug), double check your prescriptions with your doctor—sometimes using drugs this way is OK, and sometimes it isn't.

❖ Discuss with your doctor the length of time you need to take a particular drug. Some conditions require drugs indefinitely; some even require drugs for a lifetime. But you don't want to stay on anything longer than you need to.

In late 2019, Jessica Hamzelou, a reporter at *New Scientist* magazine, suggested that when medications are prescribed, we should also ask our doctors the following:

❖ How new is the drug? (New drugs may have less safety information.)

❖ Was the medicine approved for your condition? (Drugs are often prescribed "off label" for uses not yet approved by any regulatory body. It's always worth asking, "Why should I use this?")

❖ How likely is the medicine to work? How many people have to use the drug before just one person benefits? (The higher the number, the less likely the drug will help you.)

❖ And very importantly, how does the drug compare with other existing drugs?

Hamzelou also suggests you look for studies on the drug. Find out how it was approved by searching the website of a regulatory body, such as the FDA. Cochrane Reviews also provides summaries that are easy to understand on how the drug fared in clinical trials.[46]

One last thing to consider: Many popular drugs have transitioned from being by prescription only to being available over the counter. And that's an issue, because while prescription drugs are required by the Food and Drug

Administration to present "a fair balance" of benefits and risks, over-the-counter (OTC) drugs, monitored by the Federal Trade Commission, face no such requirement. As a result, it's harder for consumers to be aware of the warnings about OTC drugs and any potential side effects they may have. You should always read the small print on the labels and the package inserts. But because that information can be really complex and hard to evaluate, it's best to check with your doctor about any OTC drug you're planning to take.[47]

Moreover, we need to ensure that in our eagerness to stay healthy and retain a high quality of life, we don't do ourselves a disservice by going overboard. All drugs have benefits and limitations that may change as new information is discovered. Here's something fun that was circulated on the Internet in 1997 and 1998 that shows exactly what I mean:

Doc, I have an earache.

2000 B.C.   Here, eat this root.

1000 B.C.   That root is heathen, say this prayer.

1850 A.D.   Prayer is superstition, drink this potion.

1930   That potion is snake oil, swallow this pill.

1970   That pill is ineffective, take this antibiotic.

2000   That antibiotic is artificial, here, eat this root.[48]

CHAPTER 7

AN UNFORTUNATE HISTORY

"A House Full of Daughters is Like a Cellar Full of Sour Beer"

History, as nearly no one seems to know, is not merely something to be read. . . . On the contrary, the great force of history comes from the fact that we carry it within us, are unconsciously controlled by it in many ways, and history is literally present *in all that we do.*

—James Baldwin

B y now, you can see how sometimes, for some very good reasons, you may not get it just right when it comes to your own health.

But, as I said in the introduction, my point is *not* to blame the victim. In fact, it's just the opposite. Which is why now I would like to back up and show you the much larger, historical context that many of us have internalized and which, at times, has led us to have self-defeating tendencies—to blame ourselves, to take a back seat to others, and to decline to press our case. When you view these as part of a larger picture, you'll find they make perfect sense. The point is, we live not just in a culture but in a whole world where for centuries women were considered inferior and hysterical (and to some extent still are), our bodies so poorly designed that all we should do is stay in our place. Is it any surprise that when we don't feel well, we're inclined to ignore it, assume our illness is all in our heads, and blame ourselves for being so irresponsible that we allowed ourselves to be sick in the first place?

In case you're still skeptical, here's a highlight tour, starting in ancient Greece and ending in the medical offices of today. You'll see how women and our bodies have long been subject to misunderstanding, ignorance, superstition, and insensitivity. Be prepared: you're in for a wild ride. For thousands of years, our reproductive organs were believed to be responsible not only for all of our illnesses, but also for our weak morals, our unstable characters, and, in some cases, our

Neera Sohoni from Stanford University points out that gender bias transcends time and cultures.

A Dutch proverb declared, "A house full of daughters is like a cellar full of sour beer."

In China, daughters were referred to as "maggots in the rice."

Among the Zulus in South Africa, daughters were considered merely "weeds."[1]

evil spirits. You may not recognize yourself in the "mutilated males," the "hysterical" weaklings, and the "scum of nature" that history has sometimes made us out to be (believe it—these are actual quotes). But you'll have to admit: we've had—and we have—a lot of unfortunate preconceptions to overcome.

Ancient Greece, 800 BCE to Approximately 146 BCE

In ancient Greece, when virgins in the Greek city of Argo revolted and fled to the mountains, their "mad behavior" was blamed on their refusal to honor the phallus. It was believed that a woman without a man could be driven to madness and fall victim to "uterine melancholy."[2] As a cure, the women were urged to have sex with strong young men. The story goes that they followed these instructions (probably quite closely) and recovered their wits.

Ancient Greece considered the male body *the* perfect form. As I mentioned in the introduction, Hippocrates (460 BCE–370 BCE), the father of medicine, and his followers believed that gynecological disorders made women's bodies inherently pathological.[3] In fact, they believed there was no such thing as separate male and female bodies. There was only one body: cold, weak, and passive meant female; hot, strong, and active meant male. The boundaries between male and female were of degree, not kind.[4]

Plato viewed the womb as "an animal: voracious, predatory, appetitive, unstable, forever reducing the female into a frail and unstable creature."[5] And Aristotle thought of us as "mutilated males;" a woman's vagina was considered an inverted penis; her ovaries, shrunken female testicles; and her uterus, the female scrotum. Our organs were forced to live inside our bodies because we lacked men's vital heat.[6]

Many physicians at the time believed that a woman's uterus wandered around her body, wreaking havoc on its journey: traveling up, it created respiratory issues; traveling down, stomach and intestinal problems.[7] Sometimes doctors placed sweet-smelling substances on the vulva to coax the meandering uterus back down to its rightful home.[8] Other times, women were hung upside down so their uterus could wander back to its correct position.[9]

As if all this weren't bad enough, we also leak. Menstruation, lactation, and tears showed that women displayed a "watery, oozing physicality." That's why we're moister and flabbier than men.[10]

A man's penis, on the other hand, was considered immovable. I spent a particularly interesting morning using various search engines to check out "wandering penises," "migrating penises," and "roving penises," and I found no literature that described a penis roving around *inside* a man's body. There was plenty of evidence, however, that many a penis roved around *outside* a man's body—although I hardly needed the Internet to find that out.

According to Dr. Eva Keuls, a classics professor at the University of Minnesota, the men in ancient Athens saw us as "caged tigers waiting to break out . . . to take revenge on the male world." She says that to contain us, they implemented draconian laws to control and safeguard our chastity. For example, if a girl lost her virginity before marriage, her father could sell her into slavery. It was the reign of the phallus, and

The reign of the phallus is still with us.

In 2008, researchers examined 16,329 images from a range of textbooks from prestigious universities in Europe, the United States, and Canada. Male bodies were used three times as often as female bodies to illustrate neutral body parts.

In 2017, further research revealed that things were still not all that different.[12]

the Athenians believed that any concession to women meant their social order would collapse.[11]

These attitudes, however, led to a more positive (although still misogynistic) view of menopause. Hippocrates believed that the cessation of bleeding meant that our unruly female bodies were assimilating with the more "knowable and orderly" bodies of men. Menopause helped us become less feminine and more "manly-hearted," which was considered a vast improvement for us.[13]

The Medieval Period, Approximately the Fifth to the Fourteenth Century

Not much had changed by the Middle Ages. A woman was seen as "a body, undisciplined by mind, as a creature ruled by her internal, and particularly her sexual, organs—a disturbing force of nature."[14]

In this context, menstruation was considered not just leaky but dangerous. History professor Joan Cadden describes how in *De secretis mulierum* (*Of the Secrets of*

Women), a text from the late thirteenth or early fourteenth century, menstruation was considered so dangerous that priests needed to know whether a woman was menstruating before they took confession:

> Priests may need to know about such things when they take confession from women, but also that they may need the information to protect themselves, since menstruating women are dangerous.[15]

During the later Middle Ages, the focus shifted to God as the prime mover of disease, which, for a while at least, let women's anatomy off the hook. Sickness was considered punishment for sinning, and, in 1664, when Anne of Austria was stricken with breast cancer, she is reported to have been sure her "former vanities" caused her disease.[16]

The Renaissance, Approximately 1400–1600

Attitudes about women didn't improve much in the fifteenth century either. *I segreti delle femine*, an Italian text, describes menstrual blood as a corrosive and poisonous fluid emitted through the eyes as well as the vagina.[17]

And in 1617, Jacques Olivier wrote a misogynist tract that was republished *seventeen times*, indicating a very eager readership. Here's part of it:

You [woman] live here on earth as the world's most imperfect creature: the scum of nature, the cause of misfortune, the source of quarrels, the toy of the foolish, the plague of the wise . . . the guardian of excrement, a monster in nature.[18]

Today we read Oliver's tract as a tad extreme. But it revealed much about society's general attitude toward women at the time. Dr. Jacques Ferrand supported these beliefs, and, five years later, in a treatise on love and melancholy, *De la maladie d'amour ou mélancolie érotique*, he described women as more "passionate, witless, maniacal, and frantic from love" than men. He believed that "uterine fury" and our strong passions would lead us to experience that same "raging or madness that comes from an excessive burning desire in the womb."[19] Marriage, meaning "legitimate" sexual intercourse, was, of course, the recommended cure.

I guess you could say that at least these doctors weren't anti-sex, which many cultures are, particularly when it comes to *women* having sex. But having sex is an awfully reductive view of the causes and cures of illness. Although it's nice to be told to go make love, it's certainly not going to cure anyone's heart disease or cancer!

Before we get to the Victorian period, I want to tell you about a fascinating theory from the 1700s regarding menopausal women. It's not clear where the idea came from, but around this time, some people believed that menopause caused women to be vulnerable to spontaneous human combustion. (No, I'm not kidding.)

In the 1763 Annual Register, poor Cornelia Bandi, age sixty-two, was described as having been discovered "mysteriously reduced to soot, ash and bone in her own home. Her body was discovered as a heap of ashes, her legs and arms untouched, with fatty, foetid moisture clinging to the furniture, tapestries and walls, penetrating the drawers and dirtying the linen."[20]

The fact that, during menopause, women could burn up and be destroyed was considered nature's way of ridding the world of such horrors.

The Victorians, Approximately the 1800s

In the wildly popular semi-autobiographical short story "The Yellow Wallpaper" (1892), Charlotte Perkins Gilman, an American writer, feminist, and lecturer, describes one of the most persistent and unpleasant views of women's health in general: that it's all in our heads. Here's an excerpt:

> John [my husband] is a physician and PERHAPS (I would not say it to a living soul, of course, but this is dead paper and a great relief to my mind)— PERHAPS that is one reason I do not get well faster.

> You see, he does not believe I am sick!
> And what can one do?

> If a physician of high standing, and one's own husband, assures friends and relatives that there is really

nothing the matter with one but temporary nervous depression—a slight hysterical tendency—what is one to do?[21]

Ultimately, Perkins left her husband, moved to California, and became a noted lecturer calling for the economic independence of women. She never again retreated from society.

By this time, we had come full circle back to the idea that women were innately sick. The Victorians ignored the organ inside our head, and, according to Dr. W. W. Bliss in 1870, a woman's uterus and ovaries directed her entire personality. Any abnormality, from irritability to insanity, could be traced to some ovarian disease.[22]

Or as Dr. M. E. Dirix wrote in *Woman's Complete Guide to Health* (1869), "Thus women are treated for diseases of the stomach, liver, kidneys, heart, lungs, etc.; yet, in most instances these diseases will be found . . . to be no diseases at all, but merely the sympathetic reactions or the symptoms of one disease, namely, a disease of the womb."[23]

Some authorities believed that God had taken a uterus and simply built a woman around it. And although menstrual blood was no longer viewed as "corrosive and poisonous fluid," Havelock Ellis (1859–1939), a British doctor and sexual psychologist, perceived menstruating women to be "periodically wounded" in their most sensitive spot. He emphasized that "even in the most healthy women, a worm harmless and unperceived gnaws periodically at the roots of life."[24]

Indeed, during this era, people believed that the activity of a woman's entire reproductive cycle was so intense that it sapped her strength and (unless she was especially diligent) her morals as well. When women's brains were acknowledged, they were considered so fragile that "the intellectual force" girls expended by studying math or Latin was believed to destroy a significant number of their brain cells and decrease their fertility. And if a girl was so devoted to her education that she insisted on going to college anyway, if she survived the ordeal and actually made it to graduation, some people believed she would stop menstruating, become sterile, and develop anemia, constipation, and a host of other physical horrors.[25]

Some authorities believed menopause was equally destructive. Here's what E. J. Tilt, author of the only English book on menopause published in the nineteenth century, had to say:

> During the change of life, the nervous system is so unhinged that . . . [the disturbance] can cause normally moral women to act without principal . . . be untruthful . . . be peevish . . . even have fits of temper . . . steal . . . leave their families . . . [and] brood in melancholy [and] self-absorption.[26]

Again, in thinking derived from ancient Greece, female old age was presented as a pleasurable respite from our "worm-ridden" fertile years, but only *if* we managed to avoid the dangers of menopause—especially moral insanity, which Tilt considered its most serious condition. Tilt advised us to carefully guard our innately delicate, nurturing, and moral natures and to avoid the morally questionable activities of

During the Victorian era, the association between menopause and moral insanity was so strong that "moral insanity due to meno-pause" was often accepted as a defense in cases of shoplifting.[28]

reading novels, having sex, dancing, and going to the theater or to parties.[27]

And, of course, who can forget hysteria, that classic malady of the middle- and upper-class Victorian lady? The term even derives from the Greek word for uterus, *hysterika*. The condition was a cluster of symptoms that had no discernable organic basis and seemed to resist medical treatment. It took a variety of forms—fits, fainting, loss of voice, and loss of appetite—and many other unrelated symptoms were swept under this umbrella diagnosis.[29]

As a result, women were offered, and often requested, ovariectomies, surgical removal of the ovaries, to help resolve their "psychological problems." Men brought their wives in for surgery in order to tame their "unruly behavior."[30] According to one doctor, after castration, women were returned to their husbands "tractable," "orderly," "industrious," and "cleanly."[31]

In general, the nineteenth-century American woman was considered "frailer," "more delicate," and possessed of a "finer" nervous system than men, which made her more irritable and "prone to overstimulation and resulting exhaustion."[33]

And this belief was more than just a minor irritant: it affected the quality of our medical care. In the 1700s and 1800s, if you became ill and could afford to pay a physician, he

Hysteria was diagnosed only rarely in men. The disease existed in men, but it was given names like "neurospasmia," "spasmodic encephalitis" and "acute cerebro-pneumogastric neuropathy." Talk about diagnostic camouflage.

Men were supposed to be rational; hysteria was considered irrational. Men were supposed to have emotional control; women were considered out of control. So if a man was diagnosed with hysteria, the diagnosis questioned man's patriarchy and power by diffusing and blurring the line between the sexes.[32]

would conduct a physical examination quite differently from the one performed today. Male doctors hesitated to touch their female patients because it was considered indelicate and undignified; people felt it was simply groping in disguise.[34]

Dr. Arthur Conan Doyle (1859–1930), of Sherlock Holmes fame, described how he had to deal with a "frightful horror" of a female patient who wouldn't let him examine her chest. Apparently the woman told him, "Young doctors take such liberties, you know, my dear."[35]

Of course, that didn't justify the totally "hands-off" approach some doctors preferred. The American obstetrician Dr. Charles D. Meigs (1792–1869) attributed his hands-off approach to his patients' "preferences." He was proud, in fact, that some of his patients preferred to suffer rather than permit him to conduct a thorough examination. He wrote, "In this country . . . there are women who prefer to suffer the extremity of danger and pain rather than waive those scruples of delicacy which prevent their maladies from being explored."[36]

The good news is that, in 1816, female modesty and an embarrassing situation prompted René Laënnec (1781–1826), a surgeon in Paris, to develop the stethoscope.

Laënnec needed to listen to the heart of a young, rather stout and large-breasted female patient. Reluctant to commit the impropriety of laying his head on her breast, he rolled a notebook into a cylinder and placed one end on her chest and the other in his ear, and he was astonished to hear how much it amplified her heartbeat.

His cylinder evolved into today's stethoscope and made it possible to explore the state of internal organs before patients became cadavers, a situation of course much more useful to patients.[38]

Physician William Goodell (1829–1894), from the University of Pennsylvania, was so concerned with propriety that he instructed his students to keep their eyes fixed on the ceiling when they conducted vaginal examinations.[37] A doctor would have to literally be a Sherlock Holmes to make an accurate diagnosis under these circumstances.

Twentieth Century

As late as the twentieth century, classical psychoanalytic theory believed that when women complained about menstruation, we were rejecting our "feminine role."[39] Of course, we may have Freud to thank for that; he believed that women's "hysteria" resulted from repressed sexual needs and other erotic conflicts. Here's what J. P. Greenhill, an American gynecologist and obstetrician, wrote in the *ninth edition* (indicating an avid and enthusiastic readership) of his textbook, *Office Gynecology* (1971):

Functional amenorrhea [absence of menstruation] may occur in women who *consciously or unconsciously cannot accept womanhood* [italics mine]. This condition is commonly noted in tomboys. . . . Functional dysmenorrhea [menstrual cramps] is generally *a symptom of a personality disorder* [italics mine] even though hormonal imbalance may be present. Therefore, a thorough study of the woman's attitudes towards femininity is often necessary.[40]

That view of menstruation seems awfully antiquated, but historical ideas can be very persistent, as Natalie Angier explains in *Woman: An Intimate Geography* (1999):

The notion that menstrual blood is toxic has pervaded human thinking west to east, up to down. Given the noxious fumes they exude, menstruating women have been said to make meat go bad, wine turn sour, bread dough fall, mirrors darken, and knives become blunt.

Menstruating women have been confined to huts, to home, to anywhere but here. Orthodox Jewish men refuse the ministrations of female physicians on the chance that she might be menstruating and pollute them more profoundly than the disease from which they suffer.[41]

It's no wonder that menstruation is often referred to as "the curse."

The Museum of Menstruation (mum.org) opened in 1994 and closed in 1998. It was begun by a man named Harry Finley, a bachelor from New Jersey. As a hobby, he collected menstrual products and advertisements from around the world.

According to the museum's collection titled "Words and Expressions for Menstruation Around the World," the term "curse" may well have derived from the Irish word *curse*—pronounced "cursa"—which actually means "course," a perfectly good word for menstruation and that has no relation at all to being "cursed."

Gloria Steinem's tongue-in-cheek article "If Men Could Menstruate," published in *Ms. Magazine* in October of 1978, sums it up well. Here's part of it:

If men could menstruate, clearly menstruation would become an enviable, worthy, masculine event:

Men would brag about how long and how much.

Young boys would talk about it as the envied beginning of manhood. Gifts, religious ceremonies, family dinners, and stag parties would mark the day. . . .

There would be Paul Newman Tampons or John Wayne Maxi Pads. . . .

Menstruation would be proof that only men could serve God and country in combat ("You have to give blood to take blood").

Menopause, too, was considered a "curse" and has generated its own share of negative PR. Dr. Robert Wilson, an obstetrician and gynecologist who first practiced in Brooklyn and became successful enough to move to Park Avenue, was a key architect of its bad reputation. Dr. Wilson wrote the best-selling book *Feminine Forever* (1966), financed by Wyeth-Ayerst, which described menopause as a "staggering catastrophe" and one of the "saddest of human spectacles," and menopausal women as "castrates," "flabby," "shrunken," "dull-minded," and "desexed." He considered menopause a degenerative disease, "the end of her womanhood" that could (and "should") be prevented or cured with drugs.[42] In the description below, he makes postmenopausal women sound like perpetrators in a true crime story!

> The psychological equivalent of murder in the form of broken family relations and hatred between husband and wife is a common result of menopausal change. Medical statistics can never convey the staggering total of sheer misery inflicted upon such families—men and women alike—by menopausal side effects.[43]

Although Dr. Wilson's ideas seem extreme today, they were common at the time. In *Hot Flushes, Cold Science: A History of the Modern Menopause*, Dr. Louise Foxcroft from the University of Cambridge, quotes from Dr. David Reuben's 1969 best seller, *Everything You Always Wanted to Know About Sex*, on the subject: "As estrogen is shut off, a woman becomes as close as she can to being a man . . . having outlived their ovaries, women have outlived their usefulness as human beings."[45]

By 1975, Wyeth's product, Premarin, had become the fifth leading prescription drug in the United States. According to Nadine F. Marks, an associate professor at the University of Wisconsin–Madison, who cowrote a research paper on hormone therapy, "Even textbooks for gynecologists and obstetricians in the 1960s would explain how a woman's life could be destroyed if she didn't have estrogen in her body."[44]

Twenty-First Century

As Stacey Lewis pursued her diagnosis for what turned out, finally, to be Graves' disease, she realized just how common it is for women to be told, "It's all in your head." This is especially true for women who suffer from autoimmune diseases. In fact, it can take women up to five years and visits to five different doctors before getting an autoimmune disease accurately diagnosed.[46] That's partly because autoimmune symptoms can be hidden, partly because autoimmune symptoms frequently mimic the symptoms of other diseases, and partly because there are often no tests to help diagnose autoimmune diseases.

But diagnosing autoimmune diseases has an additional issue: a woman's own report of her symptoms is often the only evidence a doctor may have of a physical problem, and, unfortunately, some doctors dismiss our symptoms and still don't take us seriously. Sarah Ramey, the author of the wonderful book *The Lady's Handbook for Her Mysterious Illness* (2020), writes:

> There is a special suite of real and debilitating symptoms that have mistakenly come to be seen as the telltale signs of a woman who can't cope with the pressures of real life:
>
> ❖ Extreme fatigue
> ❖ Aching in the muscles and joints
> ❖ Chronic pain
> ❖ Multiple allergies
> ❖ Irritable bowels
> ❖ Frequent infections
> ❖ Endocrine problems
> ❖ Brain fog[47]

While things have improved since the days when women's ills were said to be the result of "the vapors" or "hysteria," many of us are accustomed to being told, "You're just stressed. Here, take these antidepressants." As Dr. Julie Holland, a psychiatrist in New York, puts it, "Doctors used to tell women they were being hysterical; now the code word is *stress*."[48] Stress is such a common diagnosis for women that many of us have come to believe and accept it at face value.

Although our beliefs about women have evolved from the days when we were considered second-class citizens in just about every way imaginable, we still have a long way to go before we can feel fully heard, seen, and understood. And an awareness of our unfortunate history can help make that happen. There's no question in my mind that many doctors are totally competent, hear what their patients say, and prescribe accordingly. Nevertheless, a recent issue of *New Scientist* magazine argues that the old ideas still prevail, particularly when medicine can't explain what's going on in our bodies:

It is more often women who are turned away with a shrug and told the problem is "all in your head.". . . Study after study has shown that women's medical concerns are taken less seriously than men's. Women face longer delays before getting a diagnosis, are more likely to have to return to a GP several times before being referred for investigations, and are less likely to have their condition classified as "urgent" in hospitals or to be offered certain kinds of pain relief.[49]

It has been hundreds of years, and women simply can't seem to escape the idea of the wandering uterus that meanders up to our brains, causing all sorts of peculiar conditions and behaviors. I think it's important to be aware of this unfortunate history and be sure that whatever decisions we make today and in the future don't, in some way, reinforce and perpetuate it and cause us to end up doing ourselves a disservice.

WHERE ARE THEY NOW?

Moving On

When I was a child, my parents and I would often eat dinner at my grandmother's on Sundays. I didn't know my grandmother well; in fact, my strongest memory of those Sunday dinners is the sticky plastic that covered her chairs and couches—"to keep them clean," she used to say. She also put lace doilies on the arms of the furniture, maybe for decoration, maybe to keep the plastic clean. Even as a kid, I recall thinking how strange this was. There was no sign of the cozy comfort household furnishings can offer or the personal information they can reveal.

As I researched this book, many of the women I met said their illnesses functioned much the way my grandmother's plastic did. It covered them up, buried them beneath layers of pain, fright, guilt, and shame. Illness can stick to us like plastic and obscure the women underneath. Each woman's illness erased her original sense of self and created a vacant space that she refurnished with guilt and shame, layered with doilies of depression and anger.

The shame that often accompanies illness can become so internalized that we tend to forget that the narrative is an imaginary one. Instead, we nurture and feed it with self-doubt until it's so seamless, so much a part of us, that we may not realize it's there. And shame is like garbage; it keeps piling up. It can pollute our decisions and taint them with our misperceptions about ourselves. We may end up making decisions that, under different circumstances, we might not have made and which we might later regret.

That's why, as I began thinking about this conclusion, I decided to contact some of the women I had interviewed to see how they were doing now. It had been approximately ten years since I first started working on the book, and I wanted to find out how they had fared over time. I wondered if they were still overwhelmed by the chaos and disarray they felt when we met. Had their negative feelings about themselves and their illnesses kept them from living happy, fulfilling lives?

In telling them about the progress of my book, I wanted to know how much hope I could offer readers about the odds of coming out on the other side of illness and shame. I've certainly documented women's vulnerabilities and the many ways in which we can succumb to that shame as well as the other beliefs that interfere with our healthcare. I've also offered some extensive suggestions to help women overcome these obstacles. But how good is it all if I can't show, through the power of example, that, over time, it's possible for even those struggling with the gravest of illnesses to go on to lead satisfying lives?

My own experience was reassuring. Through my research and over time, I feel that I've gained the self-confidence to stand up for myself better than I did when I agreed to my surgery so many years ago. But was my experience typical? I didn't want to be a Pollyanna about this whole thing if other women weren't able to overcome the shame and guilt they felt about becoming ill in the first place.

I'm very happy to report that my case is not unique. None of the women I contacted felt as hopeless or overwhelmed as they did when we first met. While each has chosen her own course, most have managed to move on to find new sources of satisfaction.

Desireé Daruma, for example, no longer sees her illness as a punishment and no longer blames herself for becoming ill. For her, a renewed relationship with God helped turn things around. It happened when she experienced being clinically dead for several minutes [from cardiac arrest] and then revived. She told me, "It literally took my death to teach me about life and what truly mattered. For me, it's not about religion, per se. It's about having a relationship with God. I have faith again. I've let God in. Every time I was about to give up, he came through."

She feels this relationship has helped prevent her from succumbing to the overwhelming self-pity and despair she felt when she first got sick. Even better, it's helped her fight back:

Despite the hand I was dealt, I found ways to make my experience an asset. When doctors said I'd have limitations with my hands, I took up ceramics. When they told me I'd have some vision loss after my eye surgeries, I took a drawing class. Anytime I was told that I wouldn't be able to do something, I wanted to prove them wrong. Much to my surprise, I did really well and found talents I didn't know I had.

In 2017, Desireé graduated magna cum laude with a degree in gerontology. She is working at an assisted-living facility and is heavily involved in the local lupus community. In 2016, she was at the California State Capitol with her local support group to proclaim May as Lupus Awareness Month.

For Beth Tiner, the road back from her hysterectomy and self-blame was secular. Helping others is what seems to have helped *her* heal, both physically and emotionally. Beth became a doula and, when she decided to semi-retire from being a doula, became very involved in art and journaling. Her health has improved and her energy is higher than before. She still has migraines about five times a month, but that's a lot fewer than the twenty or so she used to have. Also, her lost libido has reappeared, a development she's very happy about.

At some point, Beth developed fibromyalgia, which causes her pain and fatigue. But this time around, she's more accepting of her illness than she was before, and her desire to help others has made it easier for her to deal with this new condition. She says, "And yet I press on. The voices of self-blame, while still there, are much quieter now."

Robbie Davis-Floyd, whose daughter died on her twenty-first birthday, was able to rebound only after truly hitting bottom. In the decade following that tragedy, Robbie faced other major losses: the deaths of two very close friends, a breakup with a dearly loved fiancé who ended their relationship because he couldn't cope with her pain and depression, and the loss of her beloved house of thirty years to a fire. But what really took her down was a knee replacement. Not that it was the worst thing that happened to her; it was more like the final straw. She eventually became suicidal after giving up on any pretense that she could heal herself on her own:

> The pain in my knee was unbearable, as was the pain in my heart. I took a whole bunch of Ambien one night in a half-assed attempt at suicide, which was really a wake-up call to myself. I slept for almost two days straight, and when I woke up I called Sierra Tucson, an amazing rehab center in Arizona. I did the intake exam on the phone and was on the plane there within hours. I got it that I could no longer function without help. It was either get help or die. My diagnosis was trauma, anxiety, and depression.

Bad as things were, the support Robbie received at the center enabled her to get back on a path to health. That, plus the passage of time and a fulfilling career:

> I went through excruciating healing exercises and therapies they offered. They healed me and gave me back to myself. I feel like I literally fought my way back to happiness with the help of those marvelous therapists there, and today I cling to that happiness with all my strength.

Of course, I still miss my daughter, and I occasionally get overwhelmed by grief. Also, healing took a lot longer than those six months that my midwife friend told me about. Instead, it took ten years. But I have regained that precious and often elusive feeling called happiness, which I now experience most of the time. I am beyond grateful for that and for my remaining family and friends, and for the career in anthropology that continues to keep me fascinated and engaged with life and living.

Robbie has some hard-earned advice to women in similar straits: "We women so often feel ashamed if we are depressed. But I'm here to tell you that there is no shame in asking for help when you need it."

Other women I spoke with found solace in different ways. Despite her Sjögren's diagnosis, Margaret Adams continues her painting and has discovered a new source of intellectual stimulation in creative writing. She is currently finishing her second novel.

Susan Taylor, who suffered a serious blow to her sexuality after her hysterectomy, finds purpose in helping other women in the same situation. She teaches sexuality classes and works as a professional researcher/fact-checker for some websites.

And Stacey Lewis, who suffered from Graves' disease, is no longer suffering. Her medication has helped her to feel much better, and she is busy enjoying writing and being a mother.

These women taught me that whether an illness is temporary or chronic, and whether a treatment or surgery results in a partial or a full recovery, it's possible to go on to live a full and satisfying life.

Perhaps most important, I learned that the opposite of illness is not necessarily health; rather, it's the ability to find satisfaction in the face of what is—for some—a new reality. Over time, in that vacant space the women had originally furnished with shame and despair, they were able to develop new skills, new attitudes, and, in some cases, new and/or closer relationships.

Desireé and a friend wrote a poem about her illness that beautifully describes the resiliency I saw. It is a poignant and fitting ending for this book.

Less of Me . . . But More to Give!
by Desireé Daruma

Young and naive right from the start,
I lived my whole life with all of my heart.
I made bad choices, some I know,
Without regret, that sure will show.
I never gave up to this disease.
I went on with life just as I pleased.
Sometimes there were good days,
At most there were bad.
Yet still they're the best days I ever had.
We take for granted these simple pleasures.
Not realizing how much they're truly treasures.
We're challenged and tested so without end.
But luckily get support from our friends.

Our bodies change, and so do our souls.
So many times, there's just no control.

It's times like this that I often ask,
"Why me? Will this damn thing ever pass?"

And sure enough, just as I had doubt,
Visions of my life passed in and out.

Not then did I realize that I had mattered,
Until I heard all the hospital chatters.

"We're losing her . . ." is what I heard.
And that's when I hovered without a word.

My life was ending like a dream.
That's when I knew I'd better scream.

"No," I said, "I want to live,"
"This life of mine, you have to give!"

Then sure enough, they felt my heat.
Following that there came a beat.

I made my choice, this path to live,
Just less of me now . . . with more to give!

ACKNOWLEDGMENTS

Writing a book takes a village, and here are some of the people who lived in mine:

My very special thanks to my editor, Nan Wiener, PhD, who took a rough-and-tumble manuscript and turned it into a book. Nan, without you, this book would not have existed. You're definitely the best!

Another special thanks to all the women I met. Each one of them was incredibly gracious, open, and generous. Their only purpose in sharing their stories was to help other women. Thank you all so much. Without you, this book would not have been possible.

And special thanks also to Carole Browner, PhD, MPH, and distinguished research professor at UCLA's Jane and Terry Semel Institute for Neuroscience and Human Behavior and the Departments of Anthropology and Gender Studies, and to Robbie Davis-Floyd, PhD, adjunct professor in the Department of Anthropology at Rice University in Houston and fellow of the Society for Applied Anthropology. Carole and Robbie read and reread the manuscript, and their deep knowledge of the subject and insightful comments were invaluable.

And a great big thank-you to my writing group, Kathy Andrew, Janet Constantino-Leonard, Dr. Barbara Sapienza, Dr. Clarice Stasz, and Marsha Trent, who so patiently read each chapter again and again. Their questions, comments, and personal stories enriched the book.

Thanks to my two fabulous daughters, Lisa Serwin and Dr. Jill Kane, who read the book so many times they probably can recite it by heart. Thanks for all your willingness to keep rereading it and your wonderful comments, editing advice, and support.

And a very special thanks to my husband, Fred, who died just a few months ago. Thank you for all your love, support, advice, patience, and editing and, especially, for the wonderful dinners you cooked and cookies you baked while I was writing. There's nothing like freshly baked chocolate chip cookies to stimulate one's creativity.

Without all of you, this book would not exist.

RESOURCE DIRECTORY

On the next few pages, I've listed some websites I think you will find helpful. They offer a variety of services, so go through them one by one to see which you find most useful. Be aware, I cannot guarantee their reliability. Some were helpful to me when I wrote this book, and they may have changed since I last used them. Others I have never used but have heard about. Nevertheless, they're good places to begin your own research.

Before you begin your research, please, please, please check out the "Evaluating Internet Health Information" tutorial from the National Library of Medicine, which can be accessed here: https://medlineplus.gov/webeval/webeval. html. The tutorial offers tips on how to do your own research and evaluate the information you receive. It's also helpful to know that .edu (education) and .org (organization) sites are generally more reliable than .com (commercial) sites.

Finally, in *The Vagina Bible* (2019), Dr. Jen Gunter writes, "Don't go to a general search engine, like Google." That information, she points out, is not necessarily generated by a

medical expert. So what comes up may not be the best information. Dr. Gunter suggests that .gov sites have even better
quality information than .edu or .org or .com sites. The .gov
sites are typically curated by medical librarians.[1]

General Information

AARP
http://www.aarp.org/health/
The American Association of Retired Persons is a wonderful
resource that has a lot of information about a variety of topics.
They can help if you have questions about a condition, a
hospital, insurance, or Medicare. They also have a "drug
interaction checker," which can be very helpful for women
who take a variety of medications.

Agency for Healthcare Research and Quality
http://www.ahrq.gov/consumer
AHRQ is a federal agency whose mission is to improve the
quality, safety, efficiency, and effectiveness of healthcare for
all Americans. In English and Spanish, it has information on
conditions, diseases and treatments.

Centers for Disease Control and Prevention
http://www.cdc.gov
The CDC is a government agency that offers information
on a range of health topics. They offer information about
specific diseases, the latest health and travel alerts, and "Tips
for Healthy Living."

Cleveland Clinic

http://www.clevelandclinic.org

This nonprofit multispecialty academic medical center is similar to the Mayo Clinic (see below). Their website is a reliable source for general information.

Consumer Reports

http://www.consumerreports.org/health/home.htm

Consumer Reports rates products you might need to purchase (blood pressure monitors, fitness trackers, etc.). Some of the information is free; some you need to pay for. They have a health newsletter you can subscribe to called *Consumer Reports on Health*, and I recommend it highly.

Google

Sometimes it can be helpful to just do a search for your question, issue, or condition on Google or any other search engine. You can scroll through the results to find the most useful information. You need to be careful when you do this: some information will not be reliable, and some will be quite old. Be sure to notice the dates on the information you select. And remember, the information on Google is not necessarily generated by a medical expert.

Harvard Health

www.health.harvard.edu

This is an excellent resource for information on specific health conditions. It also publishes health reports on specific topics.

Health Central

http://www.healthcentral.com

Health Central has information about conditions and drugs. Type in the appropriate search word, or check their list of topics.

Healthfinder

healthfinder.gov

Published by the US Department of Health and Human Services, Healthfinder is another site that can help you research your diagnoses, diseases, or treatments.

Health Grades

https://www.healthgrades.com

This resource will help you check doctors, hospitals, and procedures; research what specific symptoms may mean; and double-check your diagnosis. It can help you get the right care, research your condition, and prepare for any procedures.

HealthyWomen.org

http://www.healthywomen.org

HealthyWomen.org is a nonprofit resource for women's health. Through its wide array of online and print publications, HW provides health information that, as you can tell from their name, deals with diseases and conditions applicable to women.

Mayo Clinic

www.mayoclinic.org

This organization is very similar to Cleveland Clinic and Harvard Health. Its website is an excellent source for information on specific conditions and diseases,

Medline Plus
https://www.nlm.nih.gov/
Sponsored by the National Library of Medicine and the National Institutes of Health, this fun and useful website provides extensive information about specific diseases, medical history, exhibitions, clinical trials, and more.

OB/GYN Net
http://www.obgyn.net
This online community for medical professionals provides up-to-date research on reproductive issues.

Office of Women's Health
http://www.womenshealth.gov/
This is the official website of the federal government's Office of Women's Health. They have information on women's diseases plus a lot of other material.

Our Bodies, Ourselves
http://www.ourbodiesourselves.org
Our Bodies, Ourselves, also known as the Boston Women's Health Book Collective, is a nonprofit public-interest women's health, education, advocacy, and consulting organization. They provide information about health, sexuality, and reproduction from a feminist and consumer perspective. They are excellent. I used their book for some of the information in this book, and I recommend them highly.

PLOS Medicine
http://www.plosmedicine.org
This website provides articles about the latest medical research. It publishes top-quality, peer-reviewed clinical research free to the public on a wide variety of topics.

Pub Med
www.ncbi.nlm.nih.gov/pubmed
Pub Med is developed and maintained by the National Center for Biotechnology Information at the US National Library of Medicine, located at the National Institutes of Health. Pub Med lets you search millions of journal citations and abstracts in the fields of medicine, nursing, dentistry, veterinary medicine, and the health care system. You can use it for free, and there's no charge to read the abstracts of the articles in which you are interested. More than likely, you will have to pay if you decide to download the full article. The articles are usually listed by date of publication, beginning with the most recent. It's an excellent resource for up-to-date information on the latest research.

Stanford Health Library
healthlibrary.stanford.edu
This is another general resource that provides scientifically based medical information to help you make informed decisions about your health and health care. You do not need to be a Stanford patient to use their services and resources.

Clinical Trials

CenterWatch Clinical Trials Listing Service

http://www.centerwatch.com/

According to their mission statement, CenterWatch assists patients in finding and volunteering for clinical trials. They provide information on clinical trials, specific drugs, and other essential health and educational resources. If you are interested in participating in a clinical trial, this is the site for you.

Research Match

http://www.researchmatch.org

This website, created by academic institutions around the country, pairs you with studies based on your personal profile and medical history. It brings together researchers and volunteers looking for a particular kind of trial.

Hospitals/Doctors

The Leapfrog Group

www.leapfroggroup.org

The Leapfrog Group is a hospital-reporting program that allows you to compare the safety performance of hospitals.

ProPublica Surgeon Scorecard

https://projects.propublica.org/surgeons/

This website lists death and complication rates for eight different common surgeries. Be aware that this site has not been updated since 2015.

US News and World Report: Best Hospitals
http://health.usnews.com/
This website lists the highest rated hospitals in the United States for most specialties.

Medical Tests

LabTests Medline
http://www.nlm.nih.gov/medlineplus/laboratorytests.html
This site tells you everything you want to know about any test you need to undergo. It's a service of the US National Library of Medicine and the National Institutes of Health. I found it a little easier to use than Lab Tests Online, below.

Lab Tests Online
http://www.labtestsonline.org/
Lab Tests Online is aptly named—like LabTests Medline, this site tells you everything you want to know about any test you need to undergo. It will tell you what to expect and how to interpret the results. It distinguishes between tests (such as blood cultures, for example) and screenings (such as colonoscopies).

Medication and Your Doctors

ProPublica's "Dollars for Doctors" Series
http:www.propublica.org/series/dollars-for-docs
This webpage provides extensive information about drug-company payments to doctors for lectures, consulting, advisory services, etc.

Medication Only

Askapatient.com

Askapatient reports patients' personal experiences of specific medications. Personal stories can be valuable in evaluating whether a particular medication is right for you.

Food and Drug Administration
http://www.fda.gov

Everything you ever wanted to know . . . The FDA reviews food products, medical devices, drugs, etc. It explains what GMOs are, how to interpret nutrition labels, the strengths and limitations of specific medical devices, information on the safety and availability of a variety of drugs, and much more. It's a gigantic website full of information.

The People's Pharmacy
http://www.peoplespharmacy.com

This website offers information about specific drugs as well as alternative remedies that patients may try to substitute after discussing them with their doctors.

Menstruation and Menopause

Many of the websites listed under General Information offer information on menstruation and menopause, but here are an additional two that will give you more specialized/specific information.

Feminist Women's Health Center
http://www.fwhc.org
Established in 1979, FWHC is a nonprofit organization that promotes and protects a woman's right to choose and receive reproductive healthcare. They provide abortion and reproductive health services and information.

North American Menopause Society
http://www.menopause.org
This nonprofit organization is dedicated to promoting the health and quality of life of women through an understanding of menopause.

Pregnancy and Childbirth

Childbirth Connection
http://www.childbirthconnection.org
Childbirth Connection is a core program of the National Partnership for Women and Families. It was founded in 1918 as Maternity Center Association. Its mission is to improve the quality of maternity care through research, education, advocacy, and policy. It is an excellent source for up-to-date information and resources on planning for pregnancy, labor, and birth.

International Cesarean Awareness Network (ICAN)
https://www.ican-online.org
This nonprofit organization's mission is to improve maternal-child health by preventing unnecessary cesareans through

education. It provides support for cesarean recovery and promotes vaginal birth after cesarean (VBAC).

Pregnancy.com
http://www.pregnancy.com

Pregnancy.com offers information about pregnancy as well as information about the paraphernalia needed to care for a new baby.

US Food and Drug Administration's "Women's Health Research" Page
www.fda.gov/ScienceResearch/SpecialTopics /WomensHealthResearch/

The Women's Health Research page promotes and conducts research initiatives that advance the understanding of sex differences and health conditions unique to women. Go to the search box, type in "pregnancy," and see if their topics are relevant for you. (You can, of course, use them for other conditions beside pregnancy.)

Sexual and Reproductive Health

Guttmacher Institute
http://www.guttmacher.org

The Guttmacher Institute is an excellent resource for information on sexual and reproductive health. Type in your search term, and you will see a list of articles pertaining to your search as well as their publication dates, so you can determine the age of the information. The articles can be read for free.

Planned Parenthood
www.plannedparenthood.org
This is an excellent site for information on sexual and reproductive health. Planned Parenthood has health centers across the country to help women, men, and teens acquire high-quality reproductive and sexual healthcare.

Support

Patients Like Me
http://www.patientslikeme.com
This website offers an opportunity for patients to find and share stories with other people who have their disease. According to the website, Patients Like Me is the world's largest personalized health network, with more than 650,000 people living with 2,900 conditions. Be aware that *they share your data* for scientific and marketing research.

Support Groups
To find a support group near you, type your disease or condition and the term "support groups" into any search engine. For example, if you suffer from endometriosis and want a support group, go to your search engine and type in "endometriosis support groups," plus your city and state. A list of support groups will come up.

ENDNOTES

Introduction

1. Hunt et al., "Compliance," 325; Browner and Sargent, "Engendering Medical Anthropology."
2. Barnett, "Why Do Men?"
3. Holland, "Women and Spending"; Bramwell, "Becoming Woman Wise."
4. Turris and Johnson, "Maintaining Integrity," 1467.
5. Stewart, "Women Blame Stress."
6. Elderkin-Thompson and Waitzkin, "Clinical Communication by Gender," 112.
7. Edwards, *Kingdom of the Sick*, 78.
8. Carr, Rabkin, and Skinner, "Too Many Meds?"; LaRue Huget, "Women Prescribed More Drugs."
9. Mintzes, "Ask Your Doctor," 19–20.
10. ProCon, "Should Prescription Drugs?"
11. Redford, "Make the Call," 19.
12. Redford, 19.
13. Edwards, *Kingdom of the Sick*, 20.
14. Porter, *Greatest Benefit*, 72.

Chapter 1

1. Richards, Reid, and Watt, "Victim-Blaming Revisited," 713–14.
2. DiGiacomo et al., "Caring for Others"; Hajdarevic et al., "Malignant Melanoma," 2679.
3. Sizensky, "New Survey."
4. Sizensky.
5. DiGiacomo et al., "Caring for Others."
6. Ruiz-Grossman, "This May Day."
7. Porter, "Weight of Elder Care."
8. Berman, "Women's Unpaid Work."
9. Cleveland Clinic, "Emotional Wellbeing."
10. DiGiacomo et al., "Caring for Others."
11. Hajdarevic et al., "Malignant Melanoma," 2677–79.
12. Turris and Johnson, "Maintaining Integrity," 1461–76.
13. *University of California, Berkeley Wellness Letter*, "14 Heart Healthy Steps," 1.
14. Turris and Johnson, "Maintaining Integrity," 1461.
15. Novicoff and Saleh, "Sex and Gender Disparities."
16. Hunt et al., "Compliance," 327.
17. Manteuffel et al., "Influence of Patient Sex," 117.

Chapter 2

1. *Harvard Health Letter*, "Matter of Opinion"; Newport, "Most Americans."
2. Mickle, "Women Being Misdiagnosed?"
3. Kahn, "Studies Show."
4. Kantrowitz, "Her Body."
5. HysterSisters, "Give Me a Second."
6. Russell, "Second Opinion."

7. Lichtman et al., "Symptom Recognition."

8. Van Such et al., "Diagnostic Agreement."

9. Mastroianni, "Getting Medically Misdiagnosed."

10. Johns Hopkins University School of Medicine, "Death from Misdiagnosis."

11. Mickle, "Women Being Misdiagnosed?"

12. Epstein and ProPublica, "When Evidence Says No."

13. Epstein and ProPublica.

14. Leavitt and Leavitt, *Improving Medical Outcomes*, 79–80.

15. Henig, "What's Wrong?"

16. American Autoimmune Related Diseases Association, "Women and Autoimmunity."

17. Browner and Mabel, *Neurogenetic Diagnoses*, 21.

18. *University of Michigan News*, "Second Opinion."

19. Klein, "Sex Bias"; Westervelt, "Medical Research Gender Gap."

20. *University of Leeds News*, "Heart Attacks in Women."

21. Chiaramonte and Friend, "Coronary Heart Disease Symptoms," 264.

22. Hoffmann and Tarzian, "Girl Who Cried Pain," 17, 19.

23. Edwards, *Kingdom of the Sick*, 115.

24. Groopman, *How Doctors Think*, 225.

25. *Consumer Reports on Health*, "Tough Calls," 4.

26. Chen, "Do Patients Trust Doctors?"

27. Groopman, *How Doctors Think*, 262.

28. Ingersoll and Gutfield, "Medical Mess."

29. Whiteman, "Misdiagnosed in Outpatient Clinics."

Chapter 3

1. Cleveland Clinic, "Sjögren's Syndrome."

2. Brandsborg, "Pain Following Hysterectomy."
3. Arumuga and Parthasarathy, "Migraine in Women"; Lonnee-Hoffmann and Pinas, "Effects of Hysterectomy."
4. Bakalar, "In Brief," D4.
5. Mensinger, Tylka, and Calamari, "Mechanisms Underlying Weight Status."
6. King, "Illness Attributions," 433–34.
7. Stewart, "Women Blame Stress."
8. Friedman et al., "Attribution of Blame," 354.
9. US Department of Health and Human Services' Office on Women's Health, "Lupus."
10. Klonoff and Landrine, "Culture and Gender Diversity," 414, 416.
11. Friedman et al., "Attribution of Blame," 352; Neng and Weck, "Attribution of Somatic Symptoms."
12. Eaton et al., "Invariant Dimensional Liability Model," 282; Neng and Weck, "Attribution of Somatic Symptoms."
13. Ogden, "Psychosocial Theory," 413.
14. Ehrenreich, *Bright-Sided*, 33.
15. Ehrenreich, 174.
16. Khomami, "Pressure to Stay Positive."
17. Charon, *Narrative Medicine*, 31.
18. Richards, Reid, and Watt, "Victim-Blaming Revisited," 713–14.
19. Burton and King, "Health Benefits," 158.
20. Smyth et al., "Effects of Writing."
21. Pennebaker, *Writing to Heal*; Murray, "Writing to Heal"; Burton and King, "Health Benefits," 160; Smyth et al., "Effects of Writing."

Chapter 4

1. The ancestors of Ashkenazi Jews come from southern and western Europe, unlike Sephardic Jews, whose ancestors come from Spain, Portugal, North Africa, and the Middle East. Although there is some debate about using ethnic categories in genetic research, Ashkenazi Jews are thought to have a higher prevalence of breast cancer than other women.
2. Street and Haidet, "Patients' Health Beliefs."
3. Porter, *Greatest Benefit*, 679.
4. Groopman, "Hurting All Over."
5. Sanders, "Patient Can't Explain," 16.
6. Brody, "My Story Is Broken," 81–82.
7. Freedman, "The Worst Patients," 28–30.
8. Frankel et al., "Doctor-Patient Communication."
9. Kelley et al., "Patient-Clinician Relationship."
10. Aisen, "Learning from Both Ends."
11. Roter and Hall, *Doctors Talking with Patients*, 7; *Consumer Reports on Health*, "What Exactly?," 1, 4; Hoffmann and Tarzian, "Girl Who Cried Pain," 13–27; Criado Perez, *Invisible Women*, 223; Marvel et al., "Soliciting the Patient's Agenda," 285.
12. Elderkin-Thompson and Waitzkin, "Clinical Communication by Gender," 112.
13. Elderkin-Thompson and Waitzkin, 112; Wool and Barsky, "Gender Differences in Somaticization," 449.
14. Roter and Hall, "Women Doctors."
15. Seale and Charteris-Black, "Illness Narratives," 1037, 1041.
16. Edwards, *Kingdom of the Sick*, 122; Hoffmann and Tarzian, "Girl Who Cried Pain," 16.
17. Andersson et al., "Gender Bias."

18. Chiaramonte and Friend, "Coronary Heart Disease Symptoms," 264.

19. Birdwell, Herbers, and Kroenke, "Evaluating Chest Pain," 1991–95.

20. National Fibromyalgia & Chronic Pain Association, "What Is Fibromyalgia?"

21. GfK Roper Public Affairs and Communication, "New Survey."

22. Avitzur, "Doctors' Patience," 11; Lazare, "Shame and Humiliation," 1655; Palmieri and Stern, "Doctor-Patient Relationship."

23. Dworkin-McDaniel, "Lies Women Tell"; Reddy, "'I Don't Smoke, Doc.'"

24. Lazare, "Shame and Humiliation," 1655.

25. Lazare, 1655; Palmieri and Stern, "Doctor-Patient Relationship."

26. Nowakowski, "Hope," 907.

27. Dworkin-McDaniel, "Lies Women Tell."

28. Avitzur, "Doctors' Patience," 11.

29. Gurmankin Levy et al., "Patient Nondisclosure."

30. *Consumer Reports on Health*, "What Exactly?," 1.

31. Roter and Hall, *Doctors Talking with Patients*, 7; *Consumer Reports on Health*, "What Exactly?," 1.

32. Rosato, "More Choice, More Power," 44.

33. Rhoades et al., "Speaking and Interruptions," 530.

34. Marvel et al., "Soliciting the Patient's Agenda," 285.

35. Leavitt and Leavitt, *Improving Medical Outcomes*, 2; Roter and Hall, *Doctors Talking with Patients*, 127–28.

36. Leavitt and Leavitt, *Improving Medical Outcomes*, 2.

37. Ogden, "What's in a Name?"

38. Leavitt and Leavitt, *Improving Medical Outcomes*, 2.
39. Gordon, "Physician, Hear Thyself."

Chapter 5

1. Lonnee-Hoffmann and Pinas, "Effects of Hysterectomy."
2. Johnson, "Depression after Surgery."
3. Sternberg, *Balance Within*, 2.
4. Ackerman, Nocera, and Bargh, "Incidental Haptic Sensations," 2.
5. Angier, "Abstract Thoughts?"
6. Angier.
7. Ranganathan et al., "Mental Power."
8. Kroenke and Spitzer, "Gender Differences," abstract; Page and Wessely, "Medically Unexplained Symptoms," 223; Yates and Dunayevich, "Somatoform Disorders"; Hanel et al., "Depression," abstract.
9. Kirmayer and Young, "Culture and Somatization," 420–30.
10. Magner, *History of Medicine*, 112–13.
11. *Harvard Men's Health Watch*, "Mental Side of Recovery."
12. Gouin and Kiecolt-Glaser, "Wound Healing," 81–93.
13. Sternberg, *Balance Within*, 13.
14. *Harvard Men's Health Watch*, "Mental Side of Recovery."
15. Hamzelou, "Long Life," 7.
16. *Harvard Men's Health Watch*, "Mental Side of Recovery."
17. Anderson, "Psychobiotic Revolution," 34.
18. Anderson, 36–37; Yang et al., "Regulating Intestinal Microbiota."
19. Anderson, "Psychobiotic Revolution," 36.
20. Leuchter, "Placebo Effect"; Macedo, Farré, and Baños, "Placebo Effect and Placebos," 337.

21. Macedo, Farré, and Baños, "Placebo Effect and Placebos," 337; Dold and Marton, "Placebo Effect"; Kaptchuk and Miller, "Placebo Effects in Medicine."
22. Specter, "Power of Nothing."
23. Dold and Marton, "Placebo Effect."
24. Newman, *Hippocrates' Shadow*, 144.
25. Moerman, *Meaning*, 50.
26. Stewart-Williams, "Placebo Puzzle," 199; Specter, "Power of Nothing."
27. Newman, *Hippocrates' Shadow*, 143; Specter, "Power of Nothing."
28. Stewart-Williams, "Placebo Puzzle," 199; Saxon et al., "Gender-Related Differences," abstract.
29. Moerman, "Meaning Response"; Lidstone et al., "Effects of Expectation," 403.
30. Moerman, "Meaning Response," 403; Kaptchuk and Miller, "Placebo Effects in Medicine"; Lidstone et al., "Effects of Expectation."
31. Benedetti, "Doctor's Words," 373; Newman, *Hippocrates' Shadow*, 142.
32. Vambheim and Arve Flaten, "Systematic Review."
33. Colloca, "Nocebo Effects," 44.
34. Newman, *Hippocrates' Shadow*, 142.
35. Reid, "Nocebo Effect."
36. Johnson, "Depression after Surgery."
37. Hahn, *Sickness and Healing*, 39.

Chapter 6

1. Carr, Rabkin, and Skinner, "Too Many Meds?"; *Consumer Reports*, "Is There a Cure?", 60; Frakt, "Drug Costs

So High?"; *University of California, Berkeley Wellness Letter*, "Drugstore Dilemma."

2. Carroll, "Unsung Role," B3.

3. LaRue Huget, "Women Prescribed More Drugs."

4. Sherman, "Women See Doctors More."

5. Woloshin et al., "Direct-to-Consumer Advertisements," 1141–46.

6. Smith, "Non-Disease."

7. Woloshin et al., "Direct-to-Consumer Advertisements," 1145.

8. Marx, "Forty Winks."

9. Marx; Parker, "Big Sleep."

10. Kreiner and Hunt, "Pursuit of Preventive Care," 870.

11. Kreiner and Hunt, 877.

12. *Consumer Reports*, "Pre-Disease."

13. Gawande, "Overkill," 42.

14. Gawande, 42.

15. Joyce, "Consumer Drug Ads."

16. Klara, Kim, and Ross, "Direct-to-Consumer Broadcast Advertisements," 651–58.

17. Mintzes, "Ask Your Doctor," 30, 46.

18. Mintzes, 30; Horovitz and Appleby, "Prescription Drug Costs."

19. ProCon, "Should Prescription Drugs?"

20. Llamas, "Selling Side Effects."

21. Faerber and Kreling, "False and Misleading Claims."

22. Barker, "Listening to Lyrica," 838.

23. Joyce, "Consumer Drug Ads."

24. Kaufman, "More Drug Ads."

25. Kaufman.

26. Mongiovi et al., "Characteristics of Medication Advertise-ments"; Mintzes et al., "Direct-to-Consumer Advertising."
27. McKinlay et al., "Patient Medication Requests."
28. ProCon, "Should Prescription Drugs?"
29. Scarlett and Young, "Medical Noncompliance."
30. Brody, "Not Taking Your Medicine."
31. Robeznieks, "Women Bear Greater Burden."
32. Rabin, "Drug-Dose Gender Gap."
33. Klein, "Sex Bias."
34. Carey et al., "Drugs and Medical Devices."
35. Klein, "Sex Bias."
36. *Scientific American*, "Clinical Trials Need More Diversity."
37. Carey et al., "Drugs and Medical Devices."
38. Clark and Stark, "FDA."
39. Reinberg, "Car Crash Risk."
40. Whiteman, Hogenmiller, and Fugh-Berman, "Opioid Epidemic."
41. Mazure and Fiellin, "Women and Opioids."
42. Koba, "Deadly Epidemic."
43. Gordon, "Physician, Hear Thyself," 16–17.
44. Gordon, 17.
45. Carr, Rabkin, and Skinner, "Too Many Meds?," 30.
46. Hamzelou, "Bad Medicine?," 39.
47. *University of California, Berkeley Wellness Letter*, "Drug-store Dilemma."
48. Duffin, *History of Medicine*, opening page.

Chapter 7

1. Sohoni, "Invisible Girl."
2. Tasca et al., "Women and Hysteria."

3. Porter, *Greatest Benefit*, 72.
4. King, *Hippocrates' Woman*, 7.
5. Scull, *Hysteria*, 13.
6. Criado Perez, *Invisible Women*, 196–97.
7. Duffin, *History of Medicine*, 245; Stein, "Wandering Uterus."
8. Stein, "Wandering Uterus."
9. Burton, "Calling Women 'Hysterical.'"
10. Porter, *Greatest Benefit*, 130.
11. Keuls, *Reign of the Phallus*, 4–6.
12. Criado Perez, *Invisible Women*, 197.
13. Foxcroft, *Hot Flushes*, 36–38.
14. Thomasset, "Nature of Women," 43.
15. Cadden, *Meanings of Sex Difference*, 175.
16. Garfinkel, "'This Trial,'" 78.
17. Park, *Secrets of Women*, 94.
18. Aughterson, *Renaissance Woman*, 41.
19. Arikha, *Passions and Tempers*, 162–65.
20. Foxcroft, *Hot Flushes*, 100–01.
21. Perkins Gilman, *Yellow Wallpaper*.
22. Ehrenreich and English, *For Her Own Good*, 120–21; Ehrenreich and English, *Complaints and Disorders*, 30.
23. Ehrenreich and English, *For Her Own Good*, 122.
24. Martin, *Woman in the Body*, 35.
25. Magner, *History of Medicine*, 448–49.
26. Barbre, "Meno-Boomers and Moral Guardians," 276.
27. Barbre, 276–77.
28. Barbre, 276.
29. Ehrenreich and English, *For Her Own Good*, 137.
30. Ehrenreich and English, 123–24.
31. Ehrenreich and English, *Complaints and Disorders*, 35.

32. Micale, *Hysterical Men*, 198, 207–09.

33. Walzer Leavitt, *Women and Health*, 112–13.

34. Porter, "What Is Disease?," 96.

35. Porter, *Greatest Benefit*, 676.

36. Porter, 676.

37. Porter, 676.

38. Duffin, *History of Medicine*, 195–96.

39. Munch, "Gender-Biased Diagnosing," 104.

40. Greenhill, *Office Gynecology*, 123.

41. Angier, *Woman*, 96–97.

42. Wilson, *Feminine Forever*, 30, 37, 57–59, 83; Singer and Wilson, "Menopause."

43. Wilson, *Feminine Forever*, 81.

44. Kolata and Petersen "Hormone Replacement Study."

45. Foxcroft, *Hot Flushes*, xviii.

46. Shaw, "Why Women Struggle."

47. Ramey, *Lady's Handbook*, 12.

48. Mickle, "Women Being Misdiagnosed?"

49. *New Scientist*, "Your Mind," 5.

Resource Directory

1. Gunter, *Vagina Bible*, 379–80.

BIBLIOGRAPHY

Ackerman, Joshua M., Christopher C. Nocera, and John A. Bargh. "Incidental Haptic Sensations Influence Social Judgments and Decisions." *Science* 328, no. 5986 (December 21, 2010): 1712–15. http://www.ncbi.nlm.nih.gov/pmc/articles/PMC3005631.

Aisen, Cindy Fox. "Learning from Both Ends of the Stethoscope." EurekAlert! (website). American Association for the Advancement of Science. April 9, 2007. https://www.eurekalert.org/pub_releases/2007-04/iu-lfb040907.php.

American Autoimmune Related Diseases Association. "Women and Autoimmunity" (web page). Accessed November 13, 2020. https://www.aarda.org/who-we-help/patients/women-and-autoimmunity.

Anderson, Scott C. "The Psychobiotic Revolution." *New Scientist*, September 7–13, 2019.

Andersson, J., P. Salander, M. Brandstetter-Hiltunen, E. Knutsson, and K. Hamberg. "Is It Possible to Identify Patient's

Sex When Reading Blinded Illness Narratives? An Experimental Study About Gender Bias." *International Journal of Equity Health* 7, no. 21 (July 2008).

Angier, Natalie. "Abstract Thoughts? The Body Takes Them Literally." *New York Times*, February 2, 2010.

Angier, Natalie. *Woman: An Intimate Geography*. New York: Houghton Mifflin, 1999.

Arikha, Noga. *Passions and Tempers: A History of the Humours*. New York: HarperCollins, 2007.

Arumugam, Murugesan, and Varadarajan Parthasarathy. "Increased Incidence of Migraine in Women Correlates with Obstetrics and Gynecological Surgical Procedures." *International Journal of Surgery* 22 (October 2015): 105–09. https://www.science direct.com/science/article/pii /S1743919115010973.

Aughterson, Kate, ed. *Renaissance Woman: A Sourcebook; Constructions of Femininity in England*. London: Routledge, 1995.

Avitzur, Orly. "Patients Who Try Doctors' Patience." *Consumer Reports on Health*, February 2013.

Bakalar, Nicholas. "In Brief." *New York Times*, October 18, 2019.

Barbre, Joy Webster. "Meno-Boomers and Moral Guardians." In *The Politics of Women's Bodies*, edited by Rose Weitz, 271–81. New York: Oxford University Press, 2003.

Barker, Kristin K. "Listening to Lyrica: Contested Illnesses and Pharmaceutical Determinism." *Social Science & Medicine* 73, no. 6 (September 2011): 833–42.

Barnett, Emma. "Why Do Men Still Need Women to Make Them Visit the Doctor?" *Telegraph* (London), November 5, 2012. http://www.telegraph.co.uk/women/womens-life/9655730/Why-do-men-still-need-women-to-make-them-visit-the-doctor.html.

Benedetti, Fabrizio. "How the Doctor's Words Affect the Patient's Brain." *Evaluation & the Health Professions* 25, no. 4 (December 2002): 369–86.

Berman, Jillian. "Women's Unpaid Work Is the Backbone of the American Economy." MarketWatch. Dow Jones Media Group. April 15, 2018. https://www.marketwatch.com/story/this-is-how-much-more-unpaid-work-women-do-than-men-2017-03-07.

Birdwell, Brian G., Jerome E. Herbers, and Kurt Kroenke. "Evaluating Chest Pain: The Patient's Presentation Style Alters the Physician's Diagnostic Approach." *Archives of Internal Medicine* 153, no. 17 (September 13, 1993): 1991–95.

Bond, Sarah E. "The Debate over Contraception Has an Ancient History." Forbes.com. November 7, 2017. https://www.forbes.com/sites/drsarahbond/2017/11/07/the-debate-over-contraception-has-an-ancient-history/?sh=473392d639c7.

Bramwell, Michael. *Becoming Woman Wise: Marketing Healthcare to Women.* Pharma Marketing Network. September 1, 2004. https://www.pharma-mkting.com/articles/pmn38-article03/.

Brandsborg, Birgitte. "Pain Following Hysterectomy: Epidemiological and Clinical Aspects." *Danish Medical Journal* 59, no. 1 (January 2012): B4374. https://www.ncbi.nlm.nih.gov/pubmed/22239844.

Brody, Howard. "My Story Is Broken; Can You Help Me Fix It? Medical Ethics and the Joint Construction of Narrative." *Literature and Medicine* 13, no. 1 (Spring 1994): 79–92.

Brody, Jane E. "The Cost of Not Taking Your Medicine." *New York Times*, April 18, 2017.

Browner, Carole H., and Pretoran H. Mabel. *Neurogenetic Diagnoses.* New York: Routledge, 2010.

Browner, Carole H., and Carolyn Sargent. "Engendering Medical Anthropology." In *Anthropologie de la santé et de la maladie: Perspectives internationales et enjeux contemporains*, edited by Francine Saillant and Serge Genest. Quebec: Presses de l'Université Laval, 2003.

Burton, Chad M., and Laura A. King. "The Health Benefits of Writing About Intensely Positive Experiences." *Journal of Research in Personality* 38 (2004): 150–63.

Burton, Sarah. "Calling Women 'Hysterical' Has Set Our Treatment Back Centuries." Huffington Post. March 28, 2019. https://www.huffpost.com/entry/women-hysterical -sexism-medicine_n_5c9917a2e4b057f7330e4ca9.

Cadden, Joan. *Meanings of Sex Difference in the Middle Ages.* New York: Cambridge University Press, 1993.

Carey, Jennifer L., Nathalie Nader, Peter R. Chai, Stephanie Carreiro, Matthew K. Griswold, and Katherine L. Boyle. "Drugs and Medical Devices: Adverse Events and the Impact on Women's Health." *Clinical Therpeutics* 1, no. 1 (January 2017). http://www.clinicaltherapeutics.com /article/S0149-2918%2816%2930922-5/abstract.

Carr, Teresa, Rachel Rabkin, and Ginger Skinner. "Too Many Meds? America's Love Affair with Prescription Medication." *Consumer Reports.* August 3, 2017. https://www.consumer reports.org/prescription-drugs/too-many-meds-americas -love-affair-with-prescription-medication/.

Carroll, Aaron. "The Unsung Role of the Pharmacist in Patient Health." *New York Times,* January 29, 2019.

Charon, Rita. *Narrative Medicine: Honoring the Stories of Illness*. New York: Oxford University Press, 2006.

Chen, Pauline. "Do Patients Trust Doctors Too Much?" *New York Times*, December 18, 2008. https://www.nytimes.com /2008/12/19/health/18chen.html.

Chiaramonte, Gabrielle, and Ronald Friend. "Medical Students' and Residents' Gender Bias in the Diagnosis, Treatment, and Interpretation of Coronary Heart Disease Symptoms." *Health Psychology* 25, no. 3 (March 2006): 255–66.

Clark, Daniel, and Lisa Stark. "FDA: Cut Ambien Dosage for Women." ABC News. January 10, 2013. https://abcnews .go.com/Health/fda-recommends-slashing-sleeping-pill -dosage-half-women/story?id=18182165.

Cleveland Clinic. "Emotional Wellbeing: Stress and Women" (web page). Accessed May 4, 2014. http://my.clevelandclinic .org/healthy_living/stress_management/hic_stress_and _women.aspx.

Cleveland Clinic. "Sjögren's Syndrome" (web page). Accessed December 18, 2020. https://my.clevelandclinic.org/health /diseases/4929-sjogrens-syndrome.

Colloca, Luana. "Nocebo Effects Can Make You Feel Pain." *Science* 358, no. 6359 (October 6, 2017): 44. http://science .sciencemag.org/content/358/6359/44.full.

Consumer Reports. "Is There a Cure for High Drug Prices?" July 29, 2016. https://www.consumerreports.org/drugs /cure-for-high-drug-prices/.

Consumer Reports. "You're Told You Have a 'Pre-Disease.' Here's What That Means." *Washington Post,* October 18, 2019. https://www.washingtonpost.com/health/youre-told-you -have-a-pre-disease-heres-what-that-means/2019/10/18 /a48722d0-ef92-11e9-8693-f487e46784aa-story.

Consumer Reports on Health. "Tough Calls: His and Hers." December 2007.

Consumer Reports on Health. "What Exactly Do You Mean, Doctor?" November 2004.

Criado Perez, Caroline. *Invisible Women: Data Bias in a World Designed for Men.* New York: Abrams Press, 2019.

DiGiacomo, Michelle, Patricia M. Davidson, Robert Zecchin, Kate Lamb, and John Daly. "Caring for Others, but Not Themselves: Implications for Health Care Interventions in Women with Cardiovascular Disease." *Nursing Research and Practice* (2011). http://www.ncbi.nlm.nih .gov/pmc/articles/PMC3169919.

Dold, Kirsten, and Hanna Marton. "Placebo Effect: Fake Pill, Real Power." *Women's Health,* November 14, 2011. http: //www.womenshealthmag.com/health/placebo-effect.

Duffin, Jacalyn. *History of Medicine: A Scandalously Short Introduction*. Toronto: University of Toronto Press, 1999.

Dworkin-McDaniel, Norine. "The Lies Women Tell Their Doctors." *Redbook*, September 25, 2008. https://www
.redbookmag.com/body/health-fitness/advice/a3965
/women-health-lies/.

Eaton, Nicholas R., Katherine M. Keyes, Robert F. Krueger, Steve Balsis, Andrew E. Skodol, Kristian E. Markon, Bridget F. Grant, and Deobrah S. Hasin. "An Invariant Dimensional Liability Model of Gender Differences in Mental Disorder Prevalence: Evidence from a National Sample." *Journal of Abnormal Psychology* 121, no. 1 (February 2012): 282–88.

Edwards, Laurie. *In the Kingdom of the Sick*. New York: Walker, 2013.

Ehrenreich, Barbara. *Bright-Sided: How the Relentless Promotion of Positive Thinking Has Undermined America*. New York: Henry Holt, 2009.

Ehrenreich, Barbara, and Deirdre English. *Complaints and Disorders: The Sexual Politics of Sickness*. New York: The Feminist Press at The City University of New York, 1973.

Ehrenreich, Barbara, and Deirdre English. *For Her Own Good*. New York: Doubleday, 1978.

Elderkin-Thompson, Virginia, and Howard Waitzkin. "Differences in Clinical Communication by Gender." *Journal of General Internal Medicine: Official Journal of the Society for Research and Education in Primary Care Internal Medicine* 14, no. 2 (February 1999): 112–21.

Epstein, David, and ProPublica. "When Evidence Says No, but Doctors Say Yes." *Atlantic*, February 2, 2017. https://www .theatlantic.com/health/archive/2017/02/when-evidence -says-no-but-doctors-say-yes/517368.

Faerber, Adrienne, and David H. Kreling. "Content Analysis of False and Misleading Claims in Television Advertising for Prescription and Nonprescription Drugs." *Journal of General Internal Medicine* 29, no. 1 (September 2013).

Foxcroft, Louise. *Hot Flushes, Cold Science: A History of the Modern Menopause*. London: Granta, 2009.

Frakt, Austin. "Why Are Drug Costs So High? Problem Traces to 1990s." *New York Times*, November 13, 2018.

Frankel, Richard, Jaya K. Rao, Lynda A. Anderson, and Thomas S. Inui. "Doctor-Patient Communication Has a Real Impact on Health." Science Daily. April 10, 2007. https://www .sciencedaily.com/releases/2007/04/070409144754.htm.

Freedman, David. "The Worst Patients in the World." *Atlantic*, July 2019. https://www.theatlantic.com/magazine/archive /2019/07/american-health-care-spending/590623/.

Friedman, Lois C., Catherine Romero, Richard Elledge, Jenny Chang, Mamta Kalidas, Mario F. Dulay, Garrett R. Lynch, and C. Kent Osborne. "Attribution of Blame, Self-Forgiving Attitude and Psychological Adjustment in Women with Breast Cancer." *Journal of Behavioral Medicine* 30, no. 4 (August 2007): 351–57.

Garfinkel, Susan. "'This Trial Was Sent in Love and Mercy for My Refinement': A Quaker Woman's Experience of Breast Cancer Surgery in 1814." In *Women and Health in America*, edited by Judith Walzer Leavitt, 68–90. Madison: University of Wisconsin Press, 1990.

Gawande, Atul. "Overkill." *New Yorker*, May 11, 2015.

GfK Roper Public Affairs and Communication. "New Survey Reveals Lupus Communication Gap as Many Patients Remain Silent on True Impact of Disease." GfK Roper, March 20, 2012. https://m.marketscreener.com/quote /stock/HUMAN-GENOME-SCIENCES-9544/news /Human-Genome-Sciences-NEW-SURVEY-REVEALS -LUPUS-COMMUNICATION-GAP-AS-MANY -PATIENTS-REMAIN-SILENT-ON-14227929/.

HysterSisters. "Give Me a Second." 2010. Video, 1:36. https: //www.hystersisters.com/vb2/videoshow.php?vid=452.

Gordon, Dan. "Physician, Hear Thyself." *UCLA Magazine*, January 2007. http://magazine.ucla.edu/depts/lifesigns /prescription-drugs/.

Gouin, Jean-Philippe, and Janice Kiecolt-Glaser. "The Impact of Psychological Stress on Wound Healing: Methods and Mechanisms." *Immunology and Allergy Clinics of North America* 31 (2011): 81–93.

Greenhill, J.P. *Office Gynecology*. 9th ed. Chicago: Year Book Medical Publishers, 1971.

Groopman, Jerome. *How Doctors Think*. New York: Houghton Mifflin, 2007.

Groopman, Jerome. "Hurting All Over." *New Yorker*, November 13, 2000.

Gunter, Jen. *The Vagina Bible*. New York: Citadel Press, 2019.

Gurmankin Levy, Andrea, Aaron M. Scherer, Brian J. Zikmund-Fisher, Knoll Larkin, Geoffrey D. Barnes, and Angela Fagerlin. "Prevalence of and Factors Associated with Patient Nondisclosure of Medically Relevant Information to Clinicians." *Jama Network* 1, no. 7 (2018).

Hahn, Robert. *Sickness and Healing*. New Haven, CT: Yale University Press, 1995.

Hajdarevic, S., M. Schmitt-Egenolf, C. Brulin, E. Sundbom, and A. Hornstein. "Malignant Melanoma: Gender Patterns in Care Seeking for Suspect Marks." *Journal of Clinical Nursing* 17, no. 18 (September 20, 2011): 2676–84.

Hamzelou, Jessica. "Bad Medicine?" *New Scientist*, November 30–December 6, 2019.

Hamzelou, Jessica. "The Key to a Long Life May Be Genes That Protect against Stress." *New Scientist*, October 12–18, 2019.

Hanel, G., P. Henningsen, W. Herzog, N. Sauer, R. Schaefert, J. Szecsenyi, and B. Lowe. "Depression, Anxiety, and Somatoform Disorders: Vague or Distinct Categories in Primary Care? Results from a Lage Cross-Sectional Study." *Journal of Psychosomatic Research* 67, no. 3 (September 2009): 189–97.

Harvard Health Letter. "A Matter of Opinion." October 2011. http://www.health.harvard.edu/newsletters/Harvard _Health_Letter/2011/October/a-matter-of-opinion?

Harvard Men's Health Watch. "The Mental Side of Recovery." April 2019. https://www.health.harvard.edu/mind-and -mood/the-mental-side-of-recovery.

Henig, Robin Marantz. "What's Wrong with Summer Stiers?" *New York Times Magazine*, February 18, 2009.

Hoffmann, Diane E., and Anita J. Tarzian. "The Girl Who Cried Pain: A Bias against Women in the Treatment of Pain." *Journal of Law, Medicine & Ethics* 29, no. 1 (Spring 2001): 13–27.

Holland, Stephanie. "Women and Spending" (web page). Sheconomy. Accessed November 14, 2020. http://she -conomy.com/report/marketing-to-women-quick-facts.

Horovitz, Bruce, and Julie Appleby. "Prescription Drug Costs Are Up; So Are TV Ads Promoting Them." *USA Today*, March 16, 2017. https://www.usatoday.com/ story/money/2017/03/16/prescription-drug-costs-up-tv -ads/99203878/.

Hunt, Linda M., Brigitte Jordan, Susan Irwin, and C.H. Browner. "Compliance and the Patient's Perspective: Con-trolling Symptoms in Everyday Life." *Culture, Medicine and Psychiatry* 13, no. 3 (September 1989): 315–34.

Ingersoll, Bruce, and Rose Gutfield. "Medical Mess: Implants in Jaw Joints Fail, Leaving Patients in Pain and Disfigured." *Wall Street Journal*, August 31, 1993. http://www.angelfire .com/nc/realitytx/articlesmoved/wsjarticle.html.

Johns Hopkins University School of Medicine. "A Method to Measure Diagnostic Errors Could Be Key to Pre-venting Disability and Death from Misdiagnosis." Medical Xpress. January 22, 2018. https://medicalxpress .com/news/2018-01-method-diagnostic-errors-key -disability.html.

Johnson, Jon. "Depression after Surgery: What You Need to Know." Medical News Today. Last modified August

20, 2019. https://www.medicalnewstoday.com/articles
/317616.php.

Joyce, Michael. "Consumer Drug Ads: The Harms That Come
with Pitching Lifestyle over Information." Healthnews
review.org. May 23, 2018. https://www.healthnews
review.org/2018/05/direct-to-consumer-tv-drug-ads/.

Kahn, Sieeka. "Studies Show That Women Are Diagnosed Years Later Than Men for Same Diseases." *Science
Times*, March 26, 2019. https://www.sciencetimes.com
/articles/19202/20190326/studies-show-women-diagnosed
-years-later-men-same-diseases.htm.

Kantrowitz, Barbara. "Her Body: When to Get a Second
Opinion." *Newsweek*, November 23, 2008. https://www
.newsweek.com/her-body-when-get-second-opinion-85165.

Kaptchuk, Ted J., and Franklin G. Miller. "Placebo Effects
in Medicine." *The New England Journal of Medicine* 373
(July 2, 2015): 8–9. http://www.nejm.org/doi/full/10.1056
/NEJMp1504023.

Kaufman, Joanne. "Think You're Seeing More Drug Ads on
TV? You Are, and Here's Why." *New York Times*, December
24, 2017. https://www.nytimes.com/2017/12/24/business
/media/prescription-drugs-advertising-tv.html.

Kelley, John M., Gordon Kraft-Todd, Lidia Schapira, Joe
Kossowsky, and Helen Riess. "The Influence of the

Patient-Clinician Relationship on Healthcare Outcomes: A Systemized Review and Meta-Analysis of Randomized Controlled Trials." *PLOS One* 9, no. 6 (April 9, 2014). https://journals.plos.org/plosone/article?id=10.1371/journal.pone.0094207.

Keuls, Eva C. *The Reign of the Phallus*. Berkeley: University of California Press, 1985.

Khomami, Nadia. "Pressure to Stay Positive May Be a Negative for Cancer Patients." *Guardian* (Great Britain), May 14, 2018. https://www.theguardian.com/society/2018/may/15/pressure-to-stay-positive-may-be-a-negative-for-cancer-patients-charity.

King, Helen. *Hippocrates' Woman: Reading the Female Body in Ancient Greece*. London: Routledge, 1998.

King, Rosemary. "Illness Attributions and Myocardial Infarction: The Influence of Gender and Socio-Economic Circumstances on Illness Beliefs." *Journal of Advanced Nursing* 37, no. 5 (March 2002): 431–38.

Kirmayer, Laurence J., and Allan Young. "Culture and Somatization: Clinical, Epidemiological, and Ethnographic Perspectives." *Journal of Psychosomatic Medicine* 60, no. 4 (July 1998): 420–30.

Klara, Kristina, Jeanie Kim, and Joseph S. Ross. "Direct-to-Consumer Broadcast Advertisements for Pharmaceuticals:

Off-Label Promotion and Adherence to FDA Guidelines." *Journal of Internal Medicine* 33, no. 5 (May 28, 2018): 651–58. https://link.springer.com/article/10.1007/s11606-017-4274-9.

Klein, Joanna. "Warning That Sex Bias in Animal Studies Poses a Public Health Problem." *New York Times*, May 31, 2019.

Klonoff, Elizabeth A., and Hope Landrine. "Culture and Gender Diversity in Commonsense Beliefs About the Causes of Six Illnesses." *Journal of Behavioral Medicine* 17, no. 4 (1994): 407–18.

Koba, Mark. "Deadly Epidemic: Prescription Drug Overdoses." *USA Today*, July 28, 2013. http://www.usatoday.com/story/money/business/2013/07/28/deadly-epidemic-prescription-drug-overdose/2584117/.

Kolata, Gina, and Melody Petersen. "Hormone Replacement Study A Shock to the Medical System." *New York Times*, July 10, 2002.

Kreiner, Meta J., and Linda M. Hunt. "The Pursuit of Preventive Care for Chronic Illness: Turning Healthy People into Chronic Patients." *Sociology of Health and Illness* 36, no. 6 (July 2014): 870–84.

Kroenke, K., and R. L. Spitzer. "Gender Differences in the Reporting of Physical and Somatoform Symptoms." *Psychomatic Medicine* 60, no. 2 (1998): 150–55.

LaRue Huget, Jennifer. "Women Prescribed More Drugs Than Men but Don't Always Take Them, Research Shows." *Washington Post*, March 20, 2012.

Lazare, Aaron. "Shame and Humiliation in the Medical Encounter." *Archives of Internal Medicine* 147, no. 9 (September 1987): 1653–58.

Leavitt, Jessica, and Fred Leavitt. *Improving Medical Outcomes: The Psychology of Doctor-Patient Visits.* Lanham, MD: Rowman & Littlefield, 2011.

Leuchter, Andrew. "Placebo Effect: The Power of the Mind in the Healing Process." Lecture at the UCLA Center for Health Sciences, Los Angeles, CA, May 18, 2004.

Lichtman, Judith H., Erica C. Leifheit-Limson, Emi Watanabe, Norrina B. Allen, Brian Garavalia, Linda S. Garavalia, John A. Spertus, Harlan M. Krumholz, and Leslie A. Curry. "Symptom Recognition and Healthcare Experiences of Young Women with Acute Myocardial Infarction." *Circulation: Cardiovascular Quality and Outcomes* 8, no. 2 (Supplement 1) (March 2015): S31–S38. https://www.ncbi.nlm.nih.gov /pmc/articles/PMC4801001.

Lidstone, Sarah C., Michael Schulzer, Katherine Dinelle, Edwin Mak, Vesna Sossi, Thomas J. Ruth, Raul de la Fuente -Fernandez, Anthony G. Phillips, and A. Jon Stoessi. "Effects of Expectation on Placebo-Induced Dopamine Release in Parkinson's Disease." *Archives of General*

Psychiatry 67, no. 8 (August 2010): 857–65. http://archpsyc .jamanetwork.com/article.aspx?articleid=210854.

Llamas, Michelle. "Selling Side Effects: Big Pharma's Marketing Machine." Drugwatch. Last modified July 28, 2020. https://www.drugwatch.com/featured/big-pharma -marketing/.

Lonnee-Hoffmann, Risa, and Ingrid Pinas. "Effects of Hysterectomy on Sexual Function." *Current Sexual Health Reports* 6, no. 4 (September 14, 2014): 244–51. https: //www.ncbi.nlm.nih.gov/pmc/articles/PMC4431708/.

Macedo, Ann, Magí Farré, and Josep-E Baños. "Placebo Effect and Placebos: What Are We Talking About? Some Conceptual and Historical Considerations." *European Journal of Clinical Pharmacology* 59, no. 4 (August 2003): 337–42.

Magner, Lois N. *A History of Medicine*. 2nd ed. Boca Raton, FL: Taylor & Francis Group, 2005.

Manteuffel, Marie, Sophy Williams, William Chen, Robert R. Verbrugge, Donald G. Pittman, and Amy Steinkellner. "Influence of Patient Sex and Gender on Medication Use, Adherence, and Prescribing Alignment with Guidelines." *Journal of Women's Health* 23, no. 2 (February 2014): 112–19.

Martin, Emily. *The Woman in the Body: A Cultural Analysis of Reproduction*. Boston: Beacon Press, 1992.

Marvel, M. Kim, Ronald M. Epstein, Kristine Flowers, and Howard B. Beckman. "Soliciting the Patient's Agenda." *Journal of the American Medical Association* 281, no. 3 (January 20, 1999): 283–87.

Marx, Patricia. "In Search of Forty Winks: Gizmos for a Good Night's Sleep." *New Yorker*, February 8, 2016. http://www.newyorker.com/magazine/2016/02/08/in -search-of-forty-winks.

Mastroianni, Brian. "Why Getting Medically Misdiagnosed Is More Common Than You May Think." Healthline.com. February 22, 2020. https://www.healthline.com/health -news/many-people-experience-getting-misdiagnosed.

Mazure, Carolyn M., and David A. Fiellin. "Women and Opioids: Something Different Is Happening Here." *The Lancet* 392, no. 10141 (July 7, 2018): 9–11. https://www .thelancet.com/journals/lancet/article/PIIS0140-6736(18) 31203-0/fulltext.

McKinlay, John B., Felicia Trachtenberg, Lisa D. Marceau, Jeffrey N. Katz, and Michael A. Fischer. "Effects of Patient Medication Requests on Physician Prescribing Behavior: Results of a Factorial Experiment." *Medical Care* 52, no. 4 (April 2014): 294–99.

Mensinger, Janell L., Tracy L. Tylka, and Margaret E. Calamari. "Mechanisms Underlying Weight Status and Health-care Avoidance in Women: A Study of Weight-Stigma,

Body-Related Shame and Guilt, and Healthcare Stress." *Body Image* 25 (June 25, 2018): 139–47. https://reader.elsevier.com/reader/sd/pii/S1740144517303790.

Micale, Mark S. *Hysterical Men: The Hidden History of Male Nervous Illness.* Cambridge, MA: Harvard University Press, 2008.

Mickle, Kelly. "Why Are So Many Women Being Misdiagnosed?" *Glamour*, August 11, 2017. https://www.glamour.com/story/why-are-so-many-women-being-misdiagnosed.

Mintzes, Barbara. "Ask Your Doctor: Women and Direct-to-Consumer Advertising." In *The Push to Prescribe*, edited by Anne Rochon Ford and Diane Saibil, 17–46. Toronto: Women's Press, 2010.

Mintzes, Barbara, Morris L. Barer, Richard L. Kravitz, Ken Bassett, Joel Lexchin, Arminée Kazanjian, Robert G. Evans, Richard Pan, and Stephan A. Marion. "How Does Direct-to-Consumer Advertising (DTCA) Affect Prescribing? A Survey in Primary Care Environments with and without Legal DTCA." *Canadian Medical Association Journal* 169, no. 5 (September 2, 2003): 405–12. https://www.ncbi.nlm.nih.gov/pubmed/12952801.

Moerman, Daniel. *Meaning, Medicine and the "Placebo Effect."* Cambridge: Cambridge University Press, 2002.

Moerman, Daniel. "The Meaning Response and the Ethics of Avoiding Placebos." *Evaluation and the Health Professions* 25, no. 4 (December 2002): 399–409.

Mongiovi, Jennifer, Grace Clarke Hillyer, Corey H. Basch, Danna Ethan, and Rodney Hammond. "Characteristics of Medication Advertisements Found in US Women's Fashion Magazines." *Health Promotion Perspectives* 7, no. 1 (2017): 28–33. https://www.ncbi.nlm.nih.gov/pmc/articles /PMC5209647.

Munch, Shari. "Gender-Biased Diagnosing of Women's Medical Complaints: Contributions of Feminist Thought, 1970–1995." *Women and Health* 40, no. 1 (2004): 101–21.

Murray, Bridget. "Writing to Heal." *Monitor* 33, no. 6 (June 2002): 54. http://www.apa.org/monitor/jun02/writing .aspx.

National Fibromyalgia & Chronic Pain Association. "What Is Fibromyalgia?" (web page). Accessed March 15, 2021. https://fibroandpain.org/what-is-fibromyalgia-2.

Neng, J. M., and F. Weck. "Attribution of Somatic Symptoms in Hypochondriasis." *Clinical Psychology and Psychotherapy Journal* 22, no. 2 (March–April 2015): 116–24. https:// pubmed.ncbi.nlm.nih.gov/24123559/.

Newman, David H. *Hippocrates' Shadow*. New York: Scribner, 2008.

Newport, Frank. "Most Americans Take Doctor's Advice without Second Opinion." Gallup. December 2, 2010. https://news.gallup.com/poll/145025/americans-doctor-advice -without-second-opinion.aspx.

New Scientist. "Your Mind Is the Matter." April, 6 2019.

Novicoff, Wendy M., and Khaled Saleh. "Examining Sex and Gender Disparities in Total Joint Arthroplasty." *Clinical Orthopaedics and Related Research* 469, no. 7 (July 2011): 1824–28. https://www.ncbi.nlm.nih.gov/pmc/articles/ PMC3111779/.

Nowakowski, Alexandra C. H. "Hope Is a Four-Letter Word: Riding the Emotional Rollercoaster of Illness Man- agement." *Sociology of Health and Illness* 38, no. 6 (July 2016): 899–915.

Ogden, Jane. "Psychosocial Theory and the Creation of the Risky Self." *Social Science and Medicine* 40, no. 3 (Febru- ary 1995): 409–15.

Ogden, Jane. "What's in a Name? An Experimental Study of Patients' Views of the Impact and Function of a Diagnosis." *Family Practice* 20, no. 3 (June 2003): 248–53. https://academic .oup.com/fampra/article/20/3/248/514734.

Page, L. A., and S. Wessely. "Medically Unexplained Symptoms: Exacerbating Factors in the Doctor-Patient Encounter."

Journal of the Royal Society of Medicine 96, no. 5 (2003): 223–27.

Palmieri, John J., and Theodore A. Stern. "Lies in the Doctor-Patient Relationship." *The Primary Care Companion to the Journal of Clinical Psychiatry* 11, no. 4 (2009): 163–68.

Park, Katharine. *Secrets of Women: Gender, Generation, and the Origins of Human Dissection.* New York: Zone Books, 2006.

Parker, Ian. "The Big Sleep." *New Yorker*, December 9, 2013. https://www.newyorker.com/magazine/2013/12/09 /the-big-sleep-2.

Pennebaker, James W. *Writing to Heal: A Guided Journal for Recovering from Trauma and Emotional Upheaval.* Oakland, CA: New Harbinger, 2004.

Perkins Gilman, Charlotte. *The Yellow Wallpaper.* Simon & Brown, 2011.

Porter, Eduardo. "The Weight of Elder Care on Women." *New York Times*, December 20, 2017.

Porter, Roy. *The Greatest Benefit to Mankind: A Medical History of Humanity.* New York: W.W. Norton, 1997.

Porter, Roy. "What Is Disease?" In *The Cambridge Illustrated History of Medicine*, edited by Roy Porter, 82–118. Cambridge: Cambridge University Press, 1996.

ProCon. "Should Prescription Drugs Be Advertised to Consumers?" ProCon.org. Last modified May 9, 2017. https://prescriptiondrugs.procon.org/view.answers .php?questionID=001603.

Rabin, Roni Caryn. "The Drug-Dose Gender Gap." *New York Times*, January 29, 2013.

Ramey, Sarah. *The Lady's Handbook for Her Mysterious Illness*. New York: Doubleday, 2020.

Ranganathan, Vinoth K., Vlodek Siemionow, Jing Z. Liu, Vinod Sahgal, and Guang H. Yue. "From Mental Power to Muscle Power—Gaining Strength by Using the Mind." *Neuropsychologia* 42, no. 7 (2004): 944–56. http://www.ncbi.nlm.nih .gov/pubmed/14998709.

Reddy, Sumathi. "'I Don't Smoke, Doc,' and Other Patient Lies." *Wall Street Journal*, February 18, 2013. http://www .wsj.com/articles/SB100014241278873234780045783065 10461212692.

Redford, Gabrielle. "Make the Call: Don't Miss a Beat." *AARP The Magazine*, Fabruary/March, 2012.

Reid, Brian. "The Nocebo Effect: Placebo's Evil Twin." *Washington Post*, April 30, 2002.

Reinberg, Steven. "Car Crash Risk Doubles for New Users of Sleeping Pills, Study Finds." Healthday News. June

11, 2015. https://consumer.healthday.com/sleep-disorder
-information-33/ambien-news-21/car-crash-risk-doubles
-for-new-users-of-sleeping-pills-study-finds-700334.html.

Rhoades, Donna R., Kay McFarland, W. Holmes Finch, and
Andrew O. Johnson. "Speaking and Interruptions During
Primary Care Office Visits." *Family Medicine* 33, no. 7
(July–August 2001): 528–32.

Richards, Helen, Margaret Reid, and Graham Watt. "Victim-
Blaming Revisited: A Qualitative Study of Beliefs About
Illness Causation, and Responses to Chest Pain." *Family
Practice* 20, no. 6 (2003): 711–16.

Robeznieks, Andis. "Women Bear Greater Burden of Opioid
Epidemic." American Medical Association (website).
June 27, 2017. https://wire.ama-assn.org/delivering-care
/women-bear-greater-burden-opioid-epidemic.

Rosato, Donna. "More Choice, More Power." *Consumer
Reports Magazine*, May 2020.

Roter, Debra L., and Judith A. Hall. *Doctors Talking with
Patients/Patients Talking with Doctors.* 2nd ed. Westport,
CT: Praeger, 2006.

Roter, Debra L., and Judith A. Hall. "Women Doctors Don't
Get the Credit They Deserve." *Journal of General Internal
Medicine* 30, no. 3 (March 2015): 273–274. https://www.ncbi
.nlm.nih.gov/pmc/articles/PMC4351279/.

Ruiz-Grossman, Sarah. "This May Day Don't Forget Billions of People Who Work Without Pay." Huffington Post. May 1, 2017. http://www.huffingtonpost.com/entry /may-day-international-workers-day-women-unpaid -labor_us_59075845e4b05c397680d927.

Russell, Elisabeth Schuler. "When Women Should Seek a Second Opinion." Edited by Deborah Harvey. Patient Navigator. February 8, 2011. https://patientnavigator.com /second_opinions/.

Sanders, Lisa. "When a Patient Can't Explain How She Feels." *New York Times Sunday Magazine*, July 14, 2013.

Saxon, L., A. J. Hiltunen, P. Hjemdahl, and S. Borg. "Gender-Related Differences in Response to Placebo in Benzodiazepine Withdrawal: A Single-Blind Pilot Study." *Psychopharmacology* 153, no. 2 (2001): 231–37.

Scarlett, William, and Steve Young. "Medical Noncompliance: The Most Ignored National Epidemic." *The Journal of the American Osteopathic Association* 116 (August 2016). https://doi.org/10.7556/jaoa.2016.111.

Scientific American. "Clinical Trials Need More Diversity." September 2018.

Scull, Andrew. *Hysteria: The Biography*. Oxford: Oxford University Press, 2009.

Seale, Clive, and Jonathan Charteris-Black. "The Interaction of Age and Gender in Illness Narratives." *Ageing & Society* 28 (2008).

Shaw, Gina. "Why Women Struggle to Get the Right Diagnosis." WebMD. June 8, 2018. https://www.webmd.com /women/news/20180607/why-women-are-getting -misdiagnosed.

Sherman, Neil. "Women See Doctors More Than Men." Healthday News. July 27, 2001. https://consumer.healthday .com/public-health-information-30/centers-for-disease -control-news-120/women-see-doctors-more-than -men-400589.html.

Singer, Natasha, and Duff Wilson. "Menopause, as Brought to You by Big Pharma." *New York Times*, December 13, 2009.

Sizensky, Vera. "New Survey: Moms Are Putting Their Health Last." *HealthyWomen*, March 27, 2015. https: //www.healthywomen.org/content/article/new-survey -moms-are-putting-their-health-last.

Smith, Richard. "In Search of Non-Disease." *British Medical Journal* 324, no. 7342 (April 13, 2002): 883–85.

Smyth, Joshua M., Arthur Stone, Adam Hurewitz, and Alan Kaell. "Effects of Writing About Stressful Experiences on Sympton Reduction in Patients with Asthma or

Rheumatoid Arthritis." *Journal of the American Medical Association* 281, no. 14 (1999): 1304–09. http://jama.jama network.com/article.aspx?articleid=189437.

Sohoni, Neera. "The Invisible Girl." United Nations Development Programme's *Choices Magazine*, August 1995.

Specter, Michael. "The Power of Nothing." *New Yorker*, December 12, 2011.

Stein, Elissa. "The Wandering Uterus" (web page). Wonders and Marvels. Accessed February 13, 2012. https://www.wonder sandmarvels.com/2009/12/the-wandering-uterus.html.

Steinberg, Ruth, and Linda Robinson. *Women's Sexual Health*. New York: Donald I. Fine, 1995.

Sternberg, Esther M. *The Balance Within: The Science of Connecting Health and Emotions*. New York: W.H. Freeman, 2001.

Stewart, Donna. "Women Blame Stress for Their Breast Cancer, Attribute Positive Attitude for Remission." EurekAlert! (website). American Association for the Advancement of Science. March 6, 2001. www.eurekalert.org/pub _releases/2001-03/CftA-Wbsf-0603101.php.

Stewart-Williams, S. "The Placebo Puzzle: Putting Together the Pieces." *Journal of Health Psychology* 23, no. 2 (March 2004): 198–206.

Street, Richard L., Jr., and Paul Haidet. "How Well Do Doctors Know Their Patients? Factors Affecting Physician Understanding of Patients' Health Beliefs." *Journal of General Internal Medicine* 26, no. 1 (January 2011): 21–27.

Tasca, Cecilia, Mariangela Rapetti, Mauro Giovanni Carta, and Bianca Fadda. "Women and Hysteria in the History of Mental Health." *Clinical Practice and Epidemiology in Mental Health* 8 (2012): 110–19. https://www.ncbi.nlm.nih .gov/pmc/articles/PMC3480686/.

Thomasset, Claude. "The Nature of Women." In *A History of Women in the West, Volume II, Silences of the Middle Ages*, edited by Christine Klapisch-Zuber, translated by Arthur Goldhammer, 43–69. Cambridge: Belknap Press, 1992.

Turris, Sheila A., and Joy L. Johnson. "Maintaining Integrity: Women and Treatment Seeking for the Symptoms of Potential Cardiac Illness." *Qualitative Health Research* 18, no. 11 (November 2008): 1461–76.

University of California, Berkeley Wellness Letter. "14 Heart Healthy Steps for Women." Winter 2012.

University of California, Berkeley Wellness Letter. "Drugstore Dilemma." Spring 2019.

University of Leeds News (England). "Heart Attacks in Women More Likely to Be Missed." August 30, 2016. https://www

.leeds.ac.uk/news/article/3905/heart_attacks_in_women
_more_likely_to_be_missed.

University of Michigan News (Ann Arbor). "Second Opinion
Yields Treatment Changes for Half of Patients." November
29, 2006. https://news.umich.edu/second-opinion-yields
-treatment-changes-for-half-of-patients.

US Department of Health and Human Services' Office on
Women's Health. "Lupus" (web page). Accessed March
15, 2021. https://www.womenshealth.gov/lupus.

Vambheim, Sara M., and Magne Arve Flaten. "A Systematic
Review of Sex Differences in the Placebo and the Nocebo
Effect." *Journal of Pain Research* 10 (2017): 1831–39. https:
//www.ncbi.nlm.nih.gov/pmc/articles/PMC5548268/.

Van Such, Monica, Robert Lohr, Thomas Beckman, and
James M. Naessens. "Extent of Diagnostic Agreement
among Medical Referrals." *Journal of Evaluation in
Clinical Practice* 23, no. 2 (April 2017).

Walzer Leavitt, Judith, ed. *Women and Health in America.*
2nd ed. Madison: University of Wisconsin Press, 1999.

Westervelt, Amy. "The Medical Research Gender Gap: How
Excluding Women from Clinical Trials Is Hurting Our
Health." *Guardian* (Great Britain), April 30, 2015. https:
//www.theguardian.com/lifeandstyle/2015/apr/30/fda

-clinical-trials-gender-gap-epa-nih-institute-of-medicine
-cardiovascular-disease.

Whiteman, Honor. "1 in 20 American Adults 'Misdiagnosed in Outpatient Clinics Each Year.'" Medical News Today. April 17, 2014. https://www.medicalnewstoday.com /articles/275565.php.

Whiteman, Megan, Alycia Hogenmiller, and Adriane Fugh-Berman. "Women and the Opioid Epidemic." National Women's Health Network. January 26, 2018. https://www.nwhn.org/women-opioid-epidemic/.

Wilson, Robert A. *Feminine Forever*. London: St. Anne's Press, 1966.

Woloshin, Steven, Lisa M. Schwartz, Jennifer Tremmel, and H. Gilbert Welch. "Direct-to-Consumer Advertisements for Prescription Drugs: What Are Americans Being Sold?" *The Lancet* 358 (October 6, 2001): 1141–46.

Wool, C. A., and A. J. Barsky. "Do Women Somaticize More Than Men? Gender Differences in Somatization." *Psychosomatics* 35, no. 5 (September–October 1994): 445–52.

Yang, Beibei, Jinbao Wei, Peijun Ju, and Jinghong Chen. "Effect of Regulating Intestinal Microbiota on Anxiety Symptoms: A Systematic Review." *British Medical Journal* 32, no. 2 (2019). https://gpsych.bmj.com/content/32/2/e100056.

Yates, William. "Somatic Symptom Disorders." Medscape. April 23, 2019. http://emedicine.medscape.com/article/294908.

ABOUT THE AUTHOR

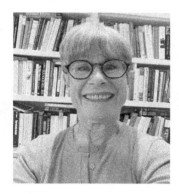

Susan Salenger was born and raised in Los Angeles, and for more than twenty-five years, Susan and her husband owned Salenger Films which produced corporate training and development films and distributed them around the world. Sue wrote the scripts and the workbooks that accompanied the films. Once her children had grown up and she had some time for herself, Sue took some anthropology classes at UCLA. Her final project for one of those classes was a study of women who had undergone hysterectomies; that study was the catalyst for this book. Sue's wonderful husband has passed away, but she has two fabulous daughters and four incredible grandchildren. They all live in Petaluma, California, and see each other often.

SELECTED TITLES FROM SHE WRITES PRESS

She Writes Press is an independent publishing company founded to serve women writers everywhere. Visit us at www.shewritespress.com.

Stay, Breathe with Me: The Gift of Compassionate Medicine by Helen Allison, RN, MSW with Irene Allison. $16.95, 978-1-63152-062-4. From the voices of the seriously ill, their families, and a specialist with a lifelong experience in caring for them comes the wisdom of a person-centered approach—one that brings heart and compassion back into health care.

The Self-Care Solution: A Modern Mother's Must-Have Guide to Health and Well-Being by Julie Burton. $16.95, 978-1-63152-068-6. Full of essential physical, emotional and relational self-care tools—and based on research by the author that includes a survey of hundreds of moms—this book is a life raft for moms who often feel like they are drowning in the sea of motherhood.

The Vitamin Solution: Two Doctors Clear the Confusion about Vitamins and Your Health by Dr. Romy Block and Dr. Arielle Levitan. $17.95, 978-1-63152-014-3. Drs. Romy Block and Arielle Levitan cut through all of the conflicting data about vitamins to provide readers with a concise, medically sound approach to vitamin use as a means of feeling better and enhancing health.

Dog as My Doctor, Cat as My Nurse: An Animal Lover's Guide to a Healthy, Happy & Extraordinary Life by Carlyn Montes De Oca. $16.95, 978-1-63152-186-7. A groundbreaking look at how dogs and cats affect, enhance, and remedy human well-being.

Role Reversal: How to Take Care of Yourself and Your Aging Parents by Iris Waichler. $16.95, 978-1-63152-091-4. A comprehensive guide for the 45 million people currently taking care of family members who need assistance because of health-related problems.